Programming Cochlear Implants

Core Clinical Concepts in Audiology

Series Editors
James W. Hall, III, PhD
Virginia Ramachandran, AuD

Basic Audiometry
Pure-Tone Audiometry and Masking
Maureen Valente, PhD
Basic Audiometry Learning Manual
Mark DeRuiter, PhD and Virginia Ramachandran, AuD

Electrodiagnostic Audiology
Objective Assessment of Hearing
James W. Hall, III, PhD and De Wet Swanepoel, PhD

Cochlear Implants
Programming Cochlear Implants
Jace Wolfe, PhD and Erin C. Schafer, PhD

Programming Cochlear Implants

Jace Wolfe, PhD
Erin C. Schafer, PhD

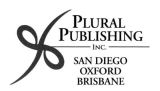

PLURAL PUBLISHING
INC.
SAN DIEGO
OXFORD
BRISBANE

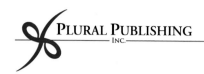

PLURAL PUBLISHING
INC.

5521 Ruffin Road
San Diego, CA 92123

e-mail: info@pluralpublishing.com
Web site: http://www.pluralpublishing.com

49 Bath Street
Abingdon, Oxfordshire OX14 1EA
United Kingdom

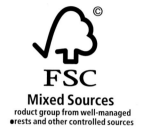

FSC
Mixed Sources
roduct group from well-managed
●rests and other controlled sources

Cert no. SW-COC-002283
www.fsc.org
© 1996 Forest Stewardship Council

Typeset in 11/13 Garamond by Flanagan's Publishing Services, Inc.
Printed in the United States of America by McNaughton and Gunn, Inc.
Second printing, September 2010

Library of Congress Cataloging-in-Publication Data

Wolfe, Jace.
 Programming cochlear implants / Jace Wolfe, Erin C. Schafer.
   p. ; cm. — (Core clinical concepts in audiology)
 Includes bibliographical references and index.
 ISBN-13: 978-1-59756-372-7 (alk. paper)
 ISBN-10: 1-59756-372-2 (alk. paper)
 1. Cochlear implants. I. Schafer, Erin C. II. Title. III. Series: Core clinical concepts in audiology.
 [DNLM: 1. Cochlear Implants. 2. Software. WV 274 W855p 2010]
 RF305.W65 2010
 617.8'82—dc22
                    2010002207

Contents

Foreword

Programming Cochlear Implants by Jace Wolfe and Erin Schafer is the introductory book for the Cochlear Implant component of the Core Clinical Concepts in Audiology. Drs. Wolfe and Schafer help demystify this complex and frequently misunderstood aspect of patient management. The book provides detailed information that will help guide both new and experienced clinicians through the process of programming all three of the currently available cochlear implant systems. An overview of programming is provided, along with manufacturer-specific considerations. The authors provide practical suggestions for patient management, ranging from the simple, such as how to optimally set up the office for efficient programming, to the more complex, such as utilization of objective measures such as neural response telemetry (NRT), neural response imaging (NRI), and electrically evoked stapedial reflex thresholds (ESRTs). Entire chapters are devoted to the use of hearing assistive technology when coupled to the speech processor (Chapter 7) and to troubleshooting the speech processor (Chapter 6). We believe that this text will be used by students as they are introduced to this complex aspect of audiology, by clinicians who are interested in understanding the complexities of cochlear implant management, as well as by clinicians who actively work with implant recipients to review, update, and improve their skills. We are pleased to provide you with this first book in the series of books on cochlear implants, and look forward to providing you with other books that will facilitate an understanding of cochlear implant technology.

Teresa A. Zwolan, PhD
Series Editor
Cochear Implant Series

Preface

Clinicians must adequately program a cochlear implant for the recipient to experience an optimal outcome. Unfortunately, at this writing, no publications have described in detail how clinicians should program contemporary cochlear implants. That changes with this book! The primary objective of this well-written book, *Programming Cochlear Implants*, is to offer practical guidance for clinicians who program cochlear implants. It represents the only book in which a detailed step-by-step process of cochlear implant programming is provided with the goal of preparing the reader to successfully program cochlear implant recipients of all ages. It also represents the first publication in which comprehensive, manufacturer-specific programming information is provided. The basics of cochlear implant programming are introduced, but the authors also expand into advanced programming techniques. Manufacturer-specific information is provided, and basic terminology is presented to assist in the illustration of the fundamentals and strategies of cochlear implant programming. Specific topics covered include basics of cochlear implant terminology and programming; clinical protocols for cochlear implant management; programming considerations for bilateral cochlear implant recipients; troubleshooting during the programming process; device-specific programming techniques; basic use of objective measures to set cochlear implant programs; use of FM and assistive listening devices with cochlear implants; and management of the difficult-to-program recipient. This book is intended for practicing clinicians who are providing or plan to provide services for cochlear implant users and also for graduate-level students.

Acknowledgments

The authors would like to express sincere gratitude to Plural Publishing Inc., with particular thanks to Sadanand Singh, Terry Zwolan, Casey Stach, and Brad Stach. We also would like to thank Stephanie Beeler and Hope Wilson Ramos, graduate students in the University of North Texas Department of Speech and Hearing Sciences AuD Program, for their outstanding and unwavering support with editing, conducting literature reviews, and creating figures and tables for this book. In addition, we offer sincere thanks to representatives from several hearing-technology manufacturers, including Christy Miller and Julie Mooneyham of Advanced Bionics Corporation; Rami Banna, Janet Clarke, Kevin Franck, Esti Nel, and Pete Arkis of Cochlear Ltd.; Jennifer Lingvai and Darla Franz of MED-EL; Christine Jones, Whitney Adamson, and Diane Hammel of Phonak; and Maureen Doty Tomasula of Oticon, for providing helpful comments and suggestions to preliminary drafts of this text and photographs for this book. We also express thanks to Sarah Florence, Clinical Audiologist at the University of North Texas, for her input on the text. Finally, and most deservedly, we would like to thank all of the cochlear implant recipients we have served. It is their motivation, courage, and success that served as the impetus behind the development of this book.

I (Jace Wolfe) also would like to thank the numerous mentors who have shaped me professionally including Richard Talbott, Stephen Painton, Michael Dennis, Francis Kuk, and last but certainly not least, Michael Grim, who selflessly and aptly shared countless hours teaching a motivated but often dense student the nuances of audiology. Additionally, I would like to thank Joanna Smith, Teresa Caraway, and Drs. Stan Baker and Mark Wood for introducing me to the world of cochlear implants and providing an excellent model of patient care for persons with cochlear implants. Also, I owe a debt of gratitude to the entire team at Hearts for Hearing for inspiring me on a daily basis to provide unlimited opportunities for persons with hearing loss. Furthermore, I would like to thank my dad, mom, and sister for instilling within me passion to live my life serving others. Finally, and most importantly, I owe a heartfelt gratitude to my loving wife Lynnette, and two children, Hayden and Harper, for the love they have shown me and the pride they have in the work I do. It is only with their support that I am able to best utilize my resources to serve persons with cochlear implants.

I (Erin Schafer) would like to express many thanks to my husband, Michael, daughter, Avery, and parents, Anne and Randy Smithson for their patience and assistance during the writing of this book. Without my family's support, this project would not have been possible. I also like to give a heartfelt thanks to Lillie Atkeisson who provides loving and nurturing care to my daughter, making my responsibilities as a working parent feasible and enjoyable. Also, appreciation is expressed to my wonderful mentors, Linda Thibodeau, Carol and Jeff Cokely, Jackie Clark, Lee Wilson, Ross Roeser, and Emily Tobey, who helped me to become a confident audiologist and assistant professor through their excellent examples of leadership and teaching. Finally, I would like to thank all of my wonderful co-workers at the University of North Texas who are supportive and encouraging every day.

This book is dedicated to all current and future recipients of cochlear implants, their families, and the hearing healthcare professionals who serve them.

1

Basic Components and Operation of a Cochlear Implant

In most cases of sensorineural hearing loss, the primary site of lesion resides within the cochlea. Cochlear hearing loss results in insufficient transduction of acoustico-mechanical energy into neural impulses at the auditory nerve. The term nerve deafness frequently is used to describe sensorineural hearing loss, but this term often is a misnomer. The auditory nerve frequently is relatively intact and functional but does not receive adequate stimulation from the cochlea. A cochlear implant is surgically inserted into the cochlea to bypass the deficient part of the auditory system and to provide direct stimulation to the auditory nerve. As a result, most people with sensorineural hearing loss respond favorably to a cochlear implant. In fact, multiple channel cochlear implants are the most successful sensory prosthetic devices in the history of medicine. Children with severe to profound hearing loss who receive an implant at an early age often develop age-appropriate spoken language (Geers, Brenner, & Davidson, 2004; Nicholas & Geers, 2007; Geers, 2004; Geers, Moog, Biedenstein, Brenner, & Hayes, 2009). Adults with post-lingual deafness who receive cochlear implants frequently achieve excellent open-set sentence recognition (i.e., 100 percent; Gifford, Shallop, and Peterson, 2008; Helms et al., 2004) and can converse over the telephone (Anderson et al., 2006).

Cochlear implants also may provide benefit to people with pathologic conditions of the auditory nerve, such as auditory neuropathy spectrum disorder and fairly significant degeneration of spiral ganglion fibers (Rance & Barker, 2008).

Success with a cochlear implant is strongly influenced by the quality of the user's program created by the audiologist. A cochlear implant program, also known as a MAP, is patient specific. The program determines how the cochlear implant will provide electrical stimulation to the auditory nerve to represent speech and environmental sounds detected by the sound processor microphone. At a fundamental level, cochlear implant programming involves the determination of stimulation levels required to restore audibility for soft sounds and achieve loudness normalization for a large range of inputs. In addition to stimulation levels, audiologists programming cochlear implants also must determine numerous other adjustable parameters to allow for optimal patient performance.

According to published research and the authors' clinical experience, recipients using inappropriate cochlear implant programs experience poor performance and outcomes (Geers et al., 2004; Wolfe & Kasulis, 2008). However, optimization of these inadequate programs often allows recipients to realize remarkably good performance. Optimum initial programming is particularly important for young children who frequently cannot provide verbal feedback about the quality of the signal they receive. Children must have consistent access to speech and environmental sounds during the first few years of life to prevent long-term delays in speech, language, and auditory development.

Although creating a cochlear implant program may seem complicated, and even intimidating, clinicians can rely on basic principles of hearing science, audiology, and aural rehabilitation/habilitation to create suitable programs for recipients. The provision of a quality program is one of the most rewarding facets of audiology, as it serves to restore the recipient's access to social, academic, and professional opportunities. The primary objective of this book's authors is to provide direction to graduate students and professionals on creating the best possible programs for cochlear implant recipients of all ages.

The chapters in this book address the basic components of cochlear implants, basic terminology of programming, basic principles of programming, manufacturer-specific programming considerations, practical clinical protocols for cochlear implant programming, troubleshooting of patient problems and complications, and the use of assistive listening devices with cochlear implants. The information in this book is applicable to almost all cochlear implant systems used in contemporary clinical settings. When manufacturer-specific information is provided, it focuses on the three manufacturers that provide cochlear implant systems in North America: Advanced Bionics Corporation, Cochlear Corporation, and MED-EL Corporation.

BASIC OPERATION OF COCHLEAR IMPLANTS

Although differences exist in hardware across manufacturers, several common components exist among all cochlear implant devices. As shown in Figure 1–1, these components include an external sound processor with a transmitting cable and electromagnetic radio frequency (RF) transmitting coil, an internal receiving coil, an internal stimulator with an electrode array, and an interface device to connect the recipient sound processor to the clinician's programming computer.

The basic operation of a cochlear implant also is similar regardless of manufacturer. The microphone of the external sound processor captures acoustic signals in the user's environment and transduces the input into an electrical signal. This electrical signal typically is sent to a preamplifier to improve the signal-to-noise ratio during transmission to the processor. The preamplifier occasionally provides a greater boost for high-frequency components of the input signal because high-frequency phonemes, such as /s/, are less intense and more susceptible to masking. Next, the signal is analyzed by a sophisticated digital signal processor in the external sound processor to classify the input according to intensity, frequency, and time domains and to convert the signal into an electrical code that will represent these features at the auditory nerve. The coded signal then is converted from a digital signal back into an electrical signal and sent to the RF coil via a transmitting cable. At the RF coil, the electrical signal is converted to an electromagnetic signal (i.e., magnetic lines of flux are created as the electrical signal travels through the transmitting coil) and transmitted via electromagnetic induction to an internal receiving coil (antenna) that is directly wired to the internal stimulator. Magnets, which are located in the center of both the external RF coil and internal receiving coil, provide adhesion of the external RF coil to the head, and align the external coil directly over the internal receiving coil. The RF signal, which is device specific, also serves as the power supply for the internal stimulator. When the magnetic lines of flux (RF) pass over the internal receiving coil, an electrical signal is induced in the internal coil and passed onto the internal stimulator. The internal stimulator, which also contains a digital signal processor, converts the electrical signal into a digital code. The processor determines the stimulation needs for the user and converts the digital code to electrical pulses based on the characteristics of the input signal and a set of rules defined by the coding strategy. The electrical pulses then are sent along the electrode lead

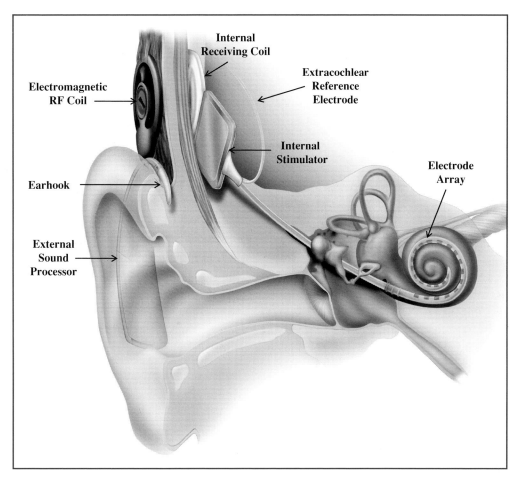

FIGURE 1–1. Basic operation of a cochlear implant. Courtesy of Cochlear™ Americas, © 2009 Cochlear Ltd.

to the stimulating intracochlear electrode contacts (Figure 1–2), where the pulses stimulate auditory nerve fibers innervating the cochlea. The electrical stimulation delivered to the intracochlear electrode contacts returns to an extracochlear electrode, which serves as the return or ground electrode (also known as the reference electrode). Extracochlear return electrodes or ground electrodes can be located on the internal device (i.e., on the case as shown in Figure 1–2) or at a location remote from the primary electrode lead (see Figure 1–1).

As previously mentioned, the electric signal from the external transmitting coil provides power to the internal device. The strength of this electric signal is adjusted on an individualized basis to minimize the necessary transmission strength and power consumption (i.e., optimize battery life). At the same time, this signal will need to provide

enough power to the internal device to stimulate and effectively represent high-level inputs, which require stronger RF strength and higher levels of stimulation.

In the most current cochlear implant systems, the external sound processor uses digital bandpass filtering, Fast Fourier transformation, or Hilbert transformation to divide the complex input signal into individual frequency segments referred to as *channels* (Figure 1–3). The output from these bandpass filters then is sent to a rectifier that captures and produces the spectral envelope (i.e., boundary across frequencies) of the input. Next, the output of the rectifier is used to modulate a train of biphasic electrical pulses (see Figure 1–3), which are delivered to the electrode contact that corresponds to a given channel. Multiple channel cochlear implants take advantage of

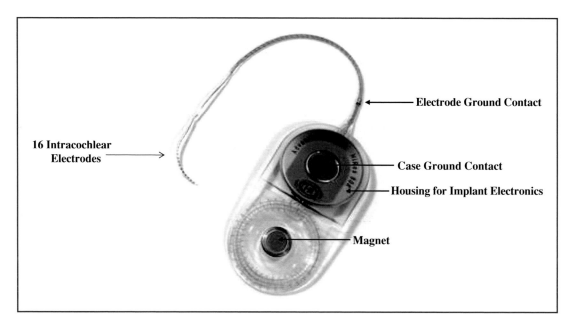

FIGURE 1–2. Advanced Bionics HiRes 90K internal stimulator and HiFocus 1j electrode. Courtesy of Advanced Bionics (http://www.AdvancedBionics.com).

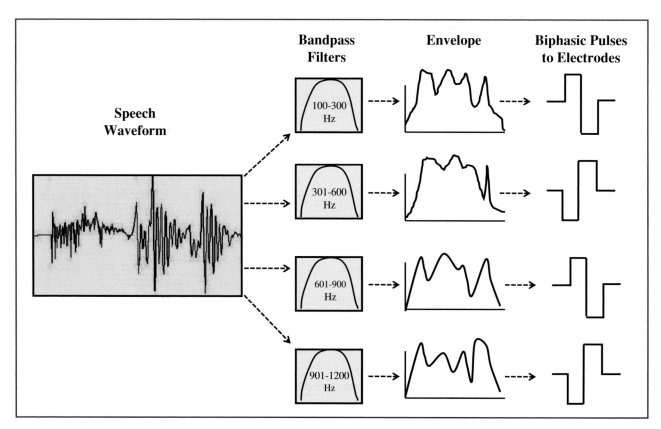

FIGURE 1–3. Diagram of how a complex signal is sent through a bandpass filter and a rectifier to determine the temporal envelope of each channel before biphasic pulses are sent to the electrode contacts.

the natural tonotopic organization of the cochlea by delivering high-frequency signals to electrodes located toward the basal end of the cochlea and low-frequency signals to more apical locations.

The power used to operate the external sound processor is delivered from a battery that is directly coupled to the sound processor. The most recent external sound processors may be operated with manufacturer- and device-specific lithium ion rechargeable batteries. This battery has several advantages over types of rechargeable batteries including a long shelf and service life, a flat voltage discharge curve, a relatively robust voltage capacity, and no memory effect. As a result, the battery does not have to be completely discharged prior to recharging it. Many sound processors also may be operated by zinc-air (similar to those used with hearing aids) or conventional alkaline batteries.

BASIC COMPONENTS OF CURRENT COCHLEAR IMPLANT SYSTEMS

Significant differences exist in the appearance and features of most current commercial sound processor for each manufacturer; however, many of the components are similar across the three manufac-turers. For instance, each sound processor contains an earhook to facilitate retention of the sound processor on the external ear, a microphone to cap-ture acoustic signals in the user's environment, a digital signal processor to analyze input signals and determine how these signals should be relayed to the user, a single power source for the sound processor and the internal device, and a transmit-ting cable and RF coil to transmit the signal to the internal device. The following sections provide details specific to the hardware of the most recently introduced cochlear implant system of each manufacturer (in alphabetical order). In addi-tion, general information on previous generations of cochlear implant systems for each manufacturer is provided in Tables 1–1 through 1–3.

Advanced Bionics Corporation

Sound Processor

The current external sound processor for the Advanced Bionics Corporation, the Harmony sound processor, is shown in Figure 1–4. The Har-mony sound processor possesses a digital signal 16-bit (96 dB) front-end processor, sampling rate of 17.4 kHz, maximum input dynamic range of

Table 1–1. Previous Internal Devices from Advanced Bionics Corporation

Device	Release Date	Description	Advantages
Clarion 1.0 & 1.2	• Clarion 1.0: 1991 for adults • Clarion 1.2: 1995, smaller version approved for pediatric trials	• Ceramic case & DSP • 16 electrodes stimulate ≤8 electrodes at once • Max stimulation rate: 1.0 is 833 pps per channel; 1.2 is 1,666 pps per channel • 3 arrays: Radial Bipolar Standard, Enhanced Bipolar, HiFocus I	• 3 coding strategies: CIS, MPS, and SAS • Case biocompatible • HiFocus array: good performance with low current levels • Telemetry system: measures electrode impedance
CII	2002	• Case similar to 1.2, device similar to HiRes 90K • Max stim rate 5000 pps per channel with PSS	• Electronics more sophisticated than 1.2 • HiRes and HiRes 120 Signal Coding

Note. CIS = continuous interleaved sampling; DSP = digital signal processor; ECAP = electrically evoked compound action potential; MPS = Multiple Pulsatile Sample; pps = pulses per second; PSS = partially simultaneous stimulation; SAS = simul-taneous analog strategy; stim = stimulation.

Table 1–2. Previous Internal Devices from Cochlear Corporation

Device	Release Date	Description	Advantages
Nucleus 24	1998	• Titanium case durable • DSP; max stim rate: 2,400 pps per channel; 14,400 pps across channels • 22 intracochlear electrode contacts • 3 arrays: Nucleus 24K Straight, Nucleus 24 Contour Advance (CA), Nucleus 24 Double Array • Telemetry: impedance & ECAP	• Durable & reliable • Supported good open-set SR • Removable magnet for MRI • Case & ball extracochlear ground electrodes; multiple electrode coupling modes • ACE, CIS, & SPEAK coding
Freedom	2005, March	• Titanium case; DSP • Max stim rate: 32,000 pps across channels; CA: 22 electrode contacts spaced variably over 15 mm • Telemetry: impedance & ECAP • 2 arrays: Contour Advance & Straight	• Durable & reliable; good open-set SR for most • Removable magnet for MRI • Case & ball extracochlear ground electrodes; multiple electrode coupling modes • Low noise floor, low stim levels for recording ECAP • ACE, CIS, & SPEAK coding

Note. ACE = advanced combination encoder; CIS = continuous interleaved sampling; ECAP = electrically-evoked compound action potential; PPS = pulses per second; SPEAK = spectral peak; SR = speech recognition; stim = stimulation.

Table 1–3. Previous Internal Devices from Med-EL Corporation

Device	Release Date	Description	Advantages
Combi 40+	Combi 40+: 2001 for adults	• Ceramic case & DSP • Max stim rate: 1,515 per channel; 18,180 pps across all channels • 12 electrodes over 30 mm, provides LF • Reference electrode: case • CIS+ coding	• Good open-set speech recognition for most • Monopolar stimulation/ electrode coupling
Pulsar CI[100]	2005	• Max stim rate: 4,225 pps per channel; 50,704 pps across channels • Most current signal coding • 24 electrode contacts in pairs; 12 electrode sites • Individual output circuits for each site	• Most current coding strategies • High rates of stim • Telemetry: electrode impedance & ECAP • Case extracochlear electrode; monopolar stim • MRI while in head at 0.2, 1.0, & 1.5 Tesla

Note. DSP = digital signal processing; CIS = continuous interleaved sampling; ECAP = electrically-evoked compound action potential; LF = low frequencies; pps = pulses per second; stim = stimulation.

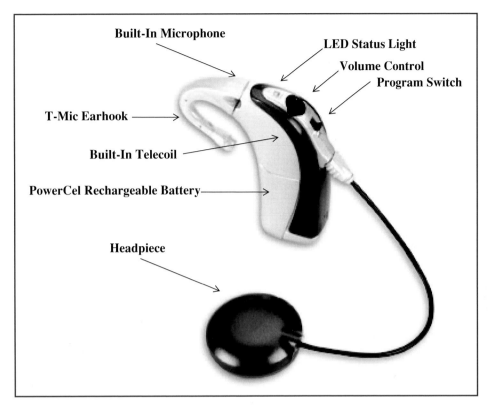

FIGURE 1–4. Advanced Bionics Harmony sound processor. Courtesy of Advanced Bionics (http://www.AdvancedBionics.com).

96 dB (i.e., maximum range of sound inputs handled without distortion), and a built-in, manually accessible telecoil. The Harmony sound processor has two user controls: (1) a rotary volume control on the dorsal-superior side of the processor and (2) a three-position slider switch just below the volume control for three distinct user programs. An LED (light emitting diode) light on the upper spine of the processor allows for troubleshooting and for indication of device status. A post at the top of the sound processor is used for coupling to specialized earhooks. The primary microphone (an omnidirectional electret microphone) of the sound processor is located at the base of this post, which also serves as an input for auxiliary signal sources.

One specialized earhook, the T-mic (see Figure 1–4), allows for auxiliary input from a small microphone located on the end of the earhook. The placement of the T-mic at the opening of the external auditory meatus creates microphone location effects that are similar to the natural ear. As such, the sound quality may be improved, and the natural directivity of the external ear is preserved. The directivity may improve speech recognition in noise, and users with bilateral cochlear implants may receive interaural timing cues. Originally, the T-mic was designed to allow for natural use of a telephone with sound from the receiver captured by the specialized microphone. In addition, many recipients use the T-mic for traditional earphone use over the auricle. Gifford & Revit, (2010) reported that recipients had significantly better speech understanding in noise in the T-mic-only mode versus the T-mic plus the primary sound processor microphone.

Other earhook options available for the Harmony sound processor include the standard, iConnect, and Direct Connect. The conventional earhook does not deliver an auxiliary signal to the sound processor and serves only to retain the device over the ear. The iConnect earhook is used to wirelessly couple a miniaturized, personal frequency modulation (FM) receiver with a three-prong Europlug connection. The Direct Connect earhook along with an accessory audio cable allows the user to connect to an MP3 player, a computer, or any other recreational audio device.

The Harmony features a socket for the headpiece. Advanced Bionics uses the term "headpiece" to describe the external transmitting cable, the transmitting coil/antenna, and the external magnet. The underside of the headpiece is available in two shapes, a flat shape (designed for use with the CII internal device) and a concave shape (designed for use with the HiRes 90K internal device) that conforms to the curvature of the head and improves retention. The magnet housed inside the headpiece allows for coupling to the receiving coil and magnet of the internal device. If the magnet strength does not allow for sufficient retention to the head, a separate magnet can

be inserted into a shallow well located on the underside of the headpiece.

As previously mentioned, the Harmony sound processor is powered by a lithium ion rechargeable battery (i.e., PowerCel). It is available in two sizes, a compact version (PowerCel Slim) and a larger version (PowerCel Plus). The former version should be suitable for all-day use for many users; however, the latter is used when more power is required to last throughout an entire day (as might be the case for recipients with exceptionally high stimulation levels, thick skin flaps, or unusually high electrode impedances). These battery packs are easily coupled to the device by sliding onto tracks located on the processor. As shown in Figure 1–5, alternative means are provided to couple the Harmony to the battery. The

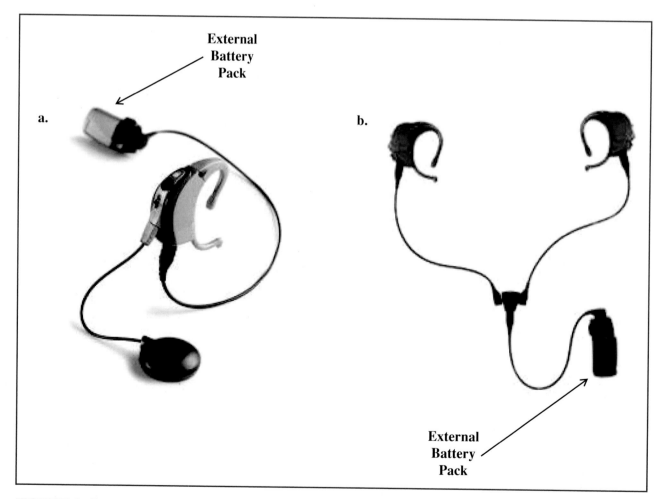

FIGURE 1–5. Advanced Bionics sound processor off-the-ear power options for (**a**) unilateral and (**b**) bilateral cochlear implant recipients. Courtesy of Advanced Bionics (http://www.AdvancedBionics.com). Pending FDA approval.

long cable (pending FDA approval) allows a person with unilateral or bilateral cochlear implants to wear the battery on his or her body, offering better retention and comfort for persons with small ears (i.e., young children). This also may be appealing for active people who play sports (pending FDA approval).

Internal Device

A picture of the Advanced Bionics HiRes 90K internal stimulator (i.e., HiRes 90K Implantable Cochlear Stimulator or ICS) and HiFocus electrode is shown in Figure 1–2. The characteristics of the Advanced Bionics HiRes 90K internal device are provided in Table 1–4. The entire internal device package is hermetically encased in a biocompatible silicone covering to prevent rejection by the human body and reduce the likelihood of bodily fluids entering the internal device. The electronics package of each internal device includes a digital signal processor that performs complex analyses on the signal received from the external sound processor and determines the magnitude of electrical stimulation for each electrode contact. The

HiRes 90K device features a digital signal processor with a sampling rate of 90,000 updates/second and a stimulation rate of 83,000 pulses/second. It has 16 independent output circuits (each with its own capacitor), which are each linked to one of the 16 individual intracochlear electrode contacts. The independent circuits allow for a high level of control over the stimulation provided to the user. The internal device also includes a bidirectional telemetry system, which enables continuous transmission of information from the external sound processor to the internal device and vice versa. The signal from the external processor is transmitted at a carrier frequency of 49 MHz, whereas the signal from the internal device is transmitted at 10.7 MHz.

The internal receiving/telemetry coil is shown in Figure 1–2 with the internal magnet positioned within a silastic sleeve in the center of the coil. The silastic sleeve permits temporary removal of the internal magnet so that the patient may undergo magnetic resonance imaging (MRI) with a strength of 1.5 Tesla. Also, a 0.3 Tesla MRI may be completed with the magnet in place. In either case, the recipient's surgeon ideally should be

Table 1–4. Characteristics of the Most Contemporary Internal Device from Each Manufacturer

Advanced Bionics: HiRes 90K	Cochlear Corporation: CI512	MED-EL Sonata TI100
• Thickness: 5.5 mm	• Thickness: 3.9 mm	• Thickness: 5.9 mm
• Fantail shaped electrode array	• Perimodiolar array	• Long array: 31.5 mm
• 16 platinum-iridium intracochlear electrodes; 2 extracochlear reference electrodes	• 22 platinum intracochlear electrodes, non-linear spacing; 2 extracochlear reference electrodes (1 on separate lead)	• 24 intracochlear concave electrodes in pairs for 12 intracochlear stimulation sites; primary and EAP reference electrodes
• Maximum stimulation rate: 83,000 pulses/second	• Maximum stimulation rate: 32,000 pulses/second	• Maximum stimulation rate: 50,704 pulses/second
• Sampling rate: 90,000 updates/second	• Telemetry system	• Telemetry system
• Telemetry system	• Coding strategies: ACE, ACE(RE), CIS, CIS(RE) & SPEAK	• Coding strategies: FSP, HD-CIS, & CIS+
• Coding strategies: HiRes-S, HiRes-P, HiRes-P/ HiRes-S Fidelity 120, MPS, & CIS	• Removable magnet for MRI up to 1.5 Tesla	• MRI safe without removal of magnet up to .2 Tesla
• Removable magnet for MRI up to 1.5 Tesla		

Note. ACE = Advanced Combination Encoder; CIS = Continuous Interleaved Sampling; FSP = Fine Structure Processing; HD = High Definition; HiRes = High Resolution; MPS = Multiple Pulsatile Sampler; MRI = Magnetic Resonance Imaging; SPEAK = Spectral Peak.

consulted prior to the procedure. The internal stimulator, which is encased in a durable, biocompatible titanium material, is positioned just below the telemetry coil. The primary reference electrode (i.e., return or ground contact) is located in the center of the casing of the internal stimulator.

Advanced Bionics uses the term "electrode array" to collectively describe the electrode lead and the electrode array. The electrode array houses the electrode contacts that ultimately provide electrical stimulation to the cochlea. The electrode lead exits the internal stimulator through a component called a feedthrough tube (not pictured). As shown, there is a fantail shape to the lead as it exits the internal stimulator, which provides flexibility and durability to the lead. The electrode lead contains 16 small wires that carry the signal from each of the 16 independent output circuits in the internal stimulator to the 16 individual electrode contacts. Medial to the fantail is a secondary return (ground) electrode referred to as the ring electrode. In rare cases, the clinician may switch the return electrode, used for stimulation from the case ground electrode, to the ring electrode. The ring electrode is also used for Neural Response Imaging (NRI) assessment. The NRI is the platform in the Advanced Bionics system used for measurement of the electrically evoked compound action potential.

The Advanced Bionics HiRes 90K internal device features two electrode choices, the HiFocus Helix electrode (Figure 1–6) and the HiFocus 1j electrode (see Figure 1–2). Both electrodes possess nonstimulating markers, which are used by the surgeon as a guide to determine how deeply to insert the electrode array. Medial to these markers are 16 platinum-iridium alloy electrode contacts numbered 1 through 16 from apex (lowest frequency) to base (highest frequency). The HiFocus electrode array has planar or "plate" electrode contacts that are positioned toward the modiolus to collectively provide a more focused delivery of stimulation to the auditory nerve.

The Helix electrode array (see Figure 1–6) has a subtly coiled shape, which is intended to facilitate close proximity of the electrode contacts to the modiolus and peripheral auditory neural elements. The most medial portion of the Helix electrode lead is thinner to allow the surgeon

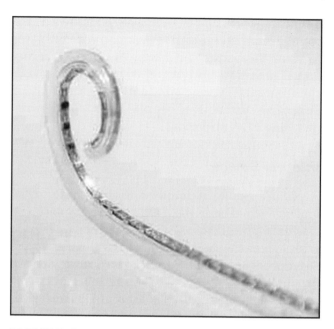

FIGURE 1–6. Advanced Bionics HiFocus internal device Helix electrode array. Courtesy of Advanced Bionics (http://www.AdvancedBionics.com).

better visualization of the cochleostomy during electrode array insertion. This type of electrode design often is referred to as a *perimodiolar* ("peri" refers to near or around the modiolous) electrode array. The theory behind a perimodiolar design is to allow for a reduction in stimulation current levels required to elicit an appropriate loudness percept for the user. However, research comparing the performance with perimodiolar Helix and the HiFocus 1j electrode arrays fails to show significant differences.

The HiFocus 1j electrode (see Figure 1–2) has a gently curved electrode array and is smaller in diameter than the Helix electrode array. Therefore, the 1j electrode permits a smaller cochleostomy for insertion. This array is most likely to be selected for a *revision surgery*, which refers to the removal of a faulty device and subsequent replacement of a new cochlear implant. After insertion of the initial electrode array, fibrous tissue may develop in and around the electrode array. As a result, when the array is removed, the channel in which it resided may be quite small in diameter. As such, the narrower diameter of the 1j facilitates an easier insertion of the replacement array. The 1j electrode array is also intended for slightly deeper insertion into the cochlea. The selection of the most appropriate electrode for a recipient often depends on the personal preference of the surgeon.

Cochlear Corporation

In September 2009, Cochlear Americas received FDA approval to commercially distribute the Nucleus 5 cochlear implant system, which includes the CP810 external sound processor (Figure 1–7), CR110 wireless remote assistant (Figure 1–8), and the CI512 internal device (Figure 1–9). The system is programmed in the CustomSound 3.0 software platform.

Sound Processor

The Nucleus CP810 (see Figure 1–7) features fully digital signal processing and three major components: (1) a cable/coil with a removable magnet, (2) a battery module, and (3) a sound processor with user controls. The sound processor also includes two omnidirectional microphones to collect acoustic inputs, a digital circuit to analyze the signal from the microphones and determine the magnitude of stimulation to be provided to the electrode contacts, and a telecoil to allow for improved hearing on the telephone and with induction loop hearing assistance technology (HAT). The CP810 is the only cochlear implant processor with an automatic telecoil to detect the presence of signals from the telephone and induction loop systems.

Furthermore, the digital processing of the CP810 is accomplished with a system known as the CHAMP-LP ASIC, which contains four separate but interrelated digital signal processors controlled by a separate digital microcontroller. The digital signal processor network possesses an asynchronous architecture that allows several different functions to occur simultaneously, but in an integrated fashion, to allow for optimal efficiency and effectiveness in signal processing. For instance, the level detector and noise management (i.e., autosensitivity) are both processing the signal at the same time to enhance efficiency, but the microcontroller evaluates the information from each processor to determine the signal output necessary to optimize signal audibility and comfort for the user. Overall, this digital signal

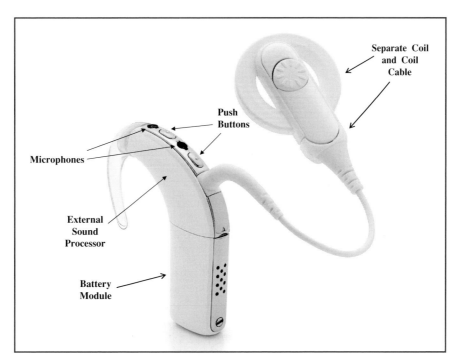

FIGURE 1–7. Cochlear Nucleus® CP810 Sound Processor. Courtesy of Cochlear™ Americas, © 2009 Cochlear Ltd.

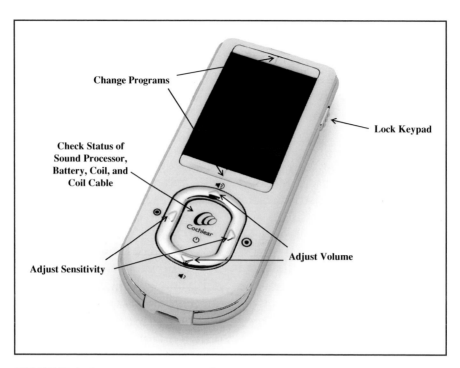

FIGURE 1–8. Cochlear Nucleus® CR110 Remote Assistant. Courtesy of Cochlear™ Americas, © 2009 Cochlear Ltd.

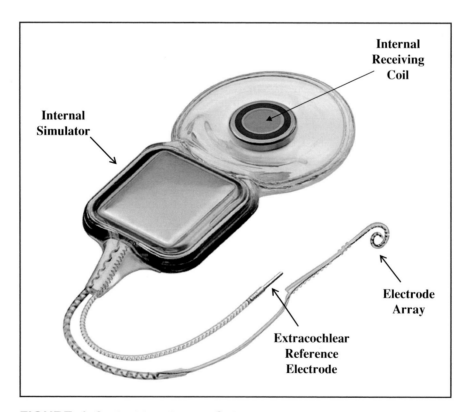

FIGURE 1–9. Cochlear Nucleus® CI512 Cochlear Implant with Contour Advance array. Courtesy of Cochlear™ Americas, © 2009 Cochlear Ltd.

processing network features 16-bit converters, with a sampling rate of 16,000 Hz and an input dynamic range of 80 dB, which in this case refers to the range between the softest sound the CP810 can detect to the most intense signal it can handle without distortion.

The CP810 sound processor is designed to be worn as an ear-level processor with a standard battery module (see Figure 1–7), but the battery module also may be attached to the sound processor via a long cable and clipped to the user's clothing via a specialized holder. This "body-worn" option, which is referred to as "Litewear," may be selected for very young children and recipients involved in sports because it minimizes the size of the unit worn on the ear. The manufacturer designed this processor to have cosmetic appeal, comfort, and good retention when worn on the ear, and it is currently the smallest external sound processor on the market. The authors' preliminary experience, as part of the third phase of an FDA-approved validation study, indicates that adult and pediatric recipients prefer the CP810 over the Nucleus Freedom (previous generation processor) in terms of comfort and retention during strenuous activity.

The battery is available in three configurations: (1) a standard, zinc-air battery module with two #675 zinc-air batteries, (2) a standard rechargeable battery module using a built-in lithium-ion battery, and (3) a smaller, compact rechargeable battery module. Tamper-proof locks are available to prevent young children from removing and potentially ingesting the battery modules or the zinc-air batteries. When using the standard, zinc-air battery module, the sound processor has a water resistance rating of IP-44. It may be splashed with water and still maintain normal function. When used with the rechargeable battery modules, the CP810 has an IP-57 rating, which means it will retain normal function after being submerged in 3 feet of water for up to 30 minutes. The processor was built on a titanium frame and features titanium connectors to couple the battery module to the sound processor. The previous processor, the Nucleus Freedom, had plastic connectors that were prone to breaking during routine "wear and tear," especially when used by active, young children. The titanium frame and connectors on the CP810 processor substantially improve the durability and reliability of this device.

The Nucleus CP810 sound processor is the only cochlear implant processor that contains two omnidirectional microphones, which allow for higher order directionality and adaptive beamforming. The two microphones are calibrated on each processor at Cochlear to account for inevitable variances that occur from microphone to microphone and subsequently allow for the desired directional response (and tighter tolerances/control of the sound quality—not just directionality, but also the amplitude-frequency response). Furthermore, the implementation of the directional system can be altered via the programming software through firmware changes. The user can select between an adaptive directional response or a very aggressive, fixed-mode response that offers substantial attenuation to sounds arriving from the sides and rear of the wearer. A removable polyester waterproof filter resides over each of the two microphones to offer protection against moisture and debris. This filter should be replaced at least every 3 months or sooner if loudness is attenuated. The processor has two push buttons for adjustments to various parameters by the recipient. The bottom button allows the recipient to power on and power off the processor with a long press and change to one of four programs with a short press. The top button may be used to manually enable or disable the built-in telecoil or activate and deactivate an accessory when connected (e.g., the personal audio cable for MP3 players). The clinician also can program the processor buttons to enable the recipient to make adjustments to the volume or the microphone sensitivity. Finally, the buttons may be locked for young children to disallow changes to the controls. A direct auditory input (DAI) accessory port is located on the spine of the processor just below the cable. This port allows for coupling to a personal FM receiver and external accessories (e.g., external microphone, MP3 cable, mains isolation cable, and monitoring earphones). The sound processor is designed to automatically recognize the connection of a DAI (and mix the signal appropriately). Additionally, the processor has a bicolor LED light at the apex of the processor underneath the removable earhook that indicates the status of the processor and the signal delivered to the internal device. The light may be deactivated, programmed to indicate the function of each button push, or programmed to alert caregivers to the status of the processor during routine use (e.g., battery life, sound detection, transmission to internal device, etc.).

The CP810 processor is designed for use with the CR110 wireless remote assistant (see Figure 1–8), permitting two-way communication between the external sound processor and the internal device. The user may adjust several settings of the sound processor including the volume, microphone sensitivity, automatic telecoil, program, telecoil and accessory- and telecoil-mixing ratios, LED light, and specificity of the directional microphone system. The remote also may be used to evaluate the status of the CP810 sound processor. The recipient or caregiver may check the battery life, the integrity of the processor, cable/coil, microphone, and radio coupling between the external and internal components. Finally, the remote assistant has an audible alarm that provides an audible warning when the status of the processor is compromised (e.g., battery is low, transmitting coil falls off of the head, etc.).

Internal Device

The Nucleus CI512 internal device (see Figure 1–9) features a sophisticated digitally driven stimulator encased in titanium. The digital signal processor of the internal device has an asynchronous architecture to enhance signal processing efficiency and effectiveness. Additional characteristics of the Cochlear Nucleus CI512 internal device are provided in Table 1–4. At the time of this writing, it is the thinnest titanium internal device available in the cochlear implant industry, making the Nucleus CI512 an appealing choice for surgeons performing cochlear implant surgery on very young children. Similar to the Advanced Bionics device, the entire internal device package is hermetically encased in biocompatible silicone.

The device has a maximum stimulation rate of 32,000 pulses per second and a digital signal processor featuring an asynchronous architecture.

This asynchronous architecture allows, among other things, the CI512 to produce stimulus pulses at any point in time rather than confining stimuli to a fixed pulse grid. This capability will allow the CI512 to execute peak-derived timing signal coding strategies, which aim to stimulate at rates consistent with the temporal fluctuations in the input signal and harbor potential for improvement of speech recognition. Additionally the CI512 has 22 stimulating leads and 22 intracochlear stimulating platinum, half-banded electrode contacts, which are positioned toward the modiolus. Similar to the other cochlear implants on the market, the CI512 has a telemetry system that facilitates two-way transmission of information from the external and internal devices. A carrier frequency of 5 MHz is used to transmit the signal in both directions. The amplifier used to record responses from the auditory nerve for diagnostic purposes has a low noise floor (less than 1 microvolt) and, as a result, enables acquisition of robust neural responses at relatively low stimulation levels.

An internal magnet is positioned within a silastic sleeve in the center of the internal receiving coil, allowing for temporary removal of the internal magnet if the patient needs an MRI. The internal stimulator is positioned just below the telemetry coil. The design of the CI512 internal device is patterned after the Nucleus Freedom internal device, which has excellent durability and reliability (<0.5 percent failure rate).

One unique characteristic of the Nucleus CI512 internal device is a reference/return electrode (known as the "Monopolar 1" or "MP1") located at the tip of a separate lead (i.e., separate from intracochlear electrode array). This arrangement permits broader stimulation fields and a reduction in the amount of current needed for a given level of stimulation. The CI512 also has an extracochlear return electrode located on the case of the stimulator (referred to as the "Monopolar 2" or "MP2"). A wide variety of stimulation modes are available and include the use of both return electrodes in isolation and in tandem, along with a special mode known as common ground stimulation (see Chapter 2).

The Nucleus CI512 provides the largest number of intracochlear stimulating electrodes (22) of all the commercially available cochlear implants.

Although it is not currently available for clinical use, it also offers dual electrode stimulation, which allows for fast, sequential stimulation of neighboring electrodes to elicit a maximum point of stimulation between two physical electrode contacts (with significantly improved battery life due to impedance drop). At the time of this writing, the CI512 has a Contour Advance array (see Figure 1–9) with a perimodiolar design and a "Softip," which is designed to reduce trauma to delicate cochlear structures during insertion. Insertion of the device using the Advanced Off-Stylet technique, along with a consistent method for identification of the cochleostomy site (just anterior and inferior to the round window), is recommended by Cochlear Ltd. These techniques reduce lateral wall force and increase the likelihood that the electrode array is not only inserted in the scala tympani, but also remains in the scala tympani throughout insertion. An emerging line of research indicates that better speech-recognition performance is associated with complete electrode insertion in the scala tympani. The electrode contacts in the Contour Advance array are spaced in a nonlinear manner to maximize the uniformity of spectral coverage for a given number of electrodes and to promote a higher probability of good speech perception.

In the future, a Straight electrode array will be available. The Straight array (an older generation electrode array) is the predecessor to the Contour Advance and is not a perimodiolar electrode. It also is thinner than the Contour and features 10 inactive stiffening rings that aid in the insertion of the array. The Straight array is recommended for patients who may have a common cavity deformity of the cochlea, fibrous tissue growth in the cochlea (i.e., bacterial meningitis), or for those undergoing revision surgery. Cochlear Ltd. also likely will offer the CI512 with a Double array electrode (at the time of this writing only available for the Nucleus 24 internal device), which possesses two electrode leads to be placed in two different cochleostomies, one in the traditional basal location and another at a more apical locale. The Double array is intended for postmeningitic recipients who have significant cochlear ossification preventing a full insertion of a conventional, single electrode array.

MED-EL Corporation

Sound Processor

The MED-EL Corporation recently introduced the OPUS 2 external sound processor for commercial use (Figure 1–10), It is small and has several enhanced features relative to previous generation processors. The OPUS 2 has a fully digital sound processor that uses a Hilbert transformation to analyze incoming acoustic inputs. It has an omnidirectional microphone located at the top of the processor just behind the earhook, an LED light that can be used to alert the user or caregiver of the processor status, and a manually accessible telecoil.

MED-EL offers several wearing options for the OPUS 2 to facilitate excellent retention and comfort for recipients with varying ear anatomy, developmental needs, and communication lifestyles. In the ear-level configuration, the OPUS 2 sound processor (see Figure 1–10) is comprised of three primary components: (1) the sound processor (i.e., control unit), (2) the angled battery pack, and (3) the cable/coil. A "connecting piece" is also required to couple the battery pack to the processor. As shown in Figure 1–11, a pediatric configuration (i.e., BabyBTE or ActiveWear) with a straight battery pack, a fixation piece, and a long cable attaching the coil to the processor allows the OPUS 2 system to be clipped to a user's clothing. This option is particularly attractive for very young children or people who play sports; however, care should be taken to position the processor microphone appropriately (i.e., toward typical sound source at 0 degrees azimuth). This option probably is not appropriate for bilaterally implanted children, where the intra-aural level differences need to be accurately maintained to help with localization. Finally, a Children's Battery Pack with a long cable connecting the battery to the sound processor allows young children to wear the processor on the ear and the battery on the body. This option removes some of the "bulk" of the device from the ear and improves the location of the processor microphone (i.e., on the ear). Tamper-proof locking features are available on the processor to prevent the child from ingesting the batteries.

The OPUS 2 is unique because it does not contain user controls on the body of the processor,

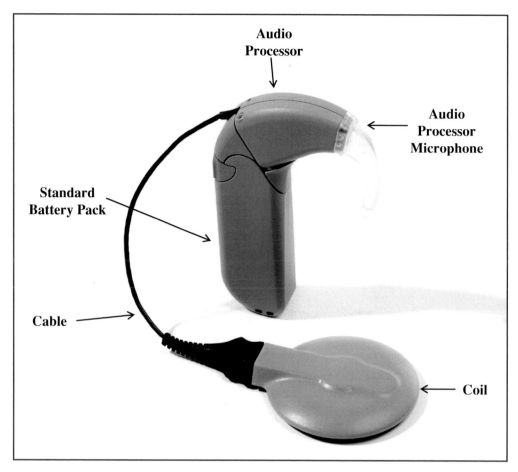

FIGURE 1–10. MED-EL Opus 2 Processor. Courtesy of MED-EL Corporation.

with the exception of a power (on/off) switch. Instead, the user may adjust the processor settings with a FineTuner remote control, which was the first remote control to be introduced in the CI industry (Figure 1–12). The FineTuner allows the recipient to adjust the volume, change the microphone sensitivity, and select up to four user programs. It also enables the user to activate the telecoil in a telecoil-only mode or a telecoil-plus-processor-microphone mode. The FineTuner can be used to make unilateral or bilateral adjustments to the processor. However, it must be synchronized to one or both processors for control via the remote.

Another novel aspect to this processor is the OPUS 2 FM Battery Pack Cover with a three-pin Europlug socket. When this battery cover is in use, the socket is located at the base of the processor. It enables wireless coupling of a personal FM receiver to the processor, or a special audio cable may be used to connect cell phones, MP3 players, laptop computers, televisions, gaming systems, and Bluetooth devices. The OPUS 2 has a variety of battery options. The recently introduced ear-level DaCapo Rechargeable Battery System (Figure 1–13) provides the user with 10 to 12 hours of operation. The processor also may be powered with three #675 zinc-air batteries (for 3 to 5 full days of battery life) or a remote battery pack utilizing one AA alkaline battery.

Internal Device

The SONATA$_{TI}$^{100} is the first MED-EL internal device encased in titanium with a silicone covering over the receiving coil (Figure 1–14). Previous internal devices were encased in a ceramic shell.

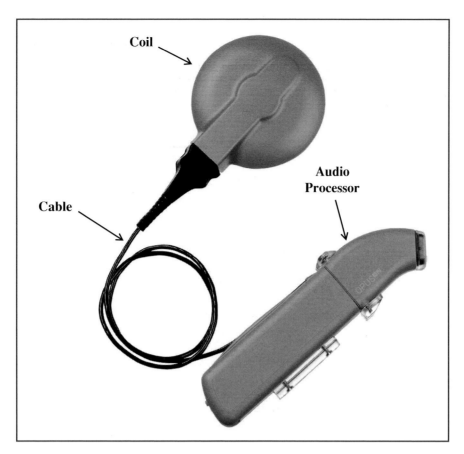

FIGURE 1–11. MED-EL Opus 2 BabyBTE option. Courtesy of MED-EL Corporation.

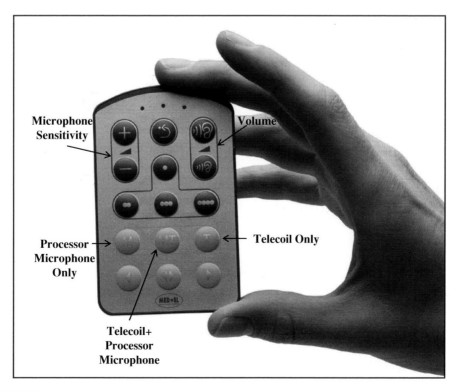

FIGURE 1–12. MED-EL FineTuner remote control. Courtesy of MED-EL Corporation.

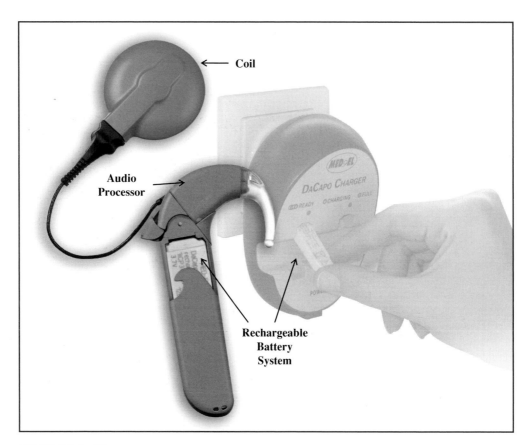

FIGURE 1–13. MED-EL DaCapo Rechargeable Battery System. Courtesy of MED-EL Corporation.

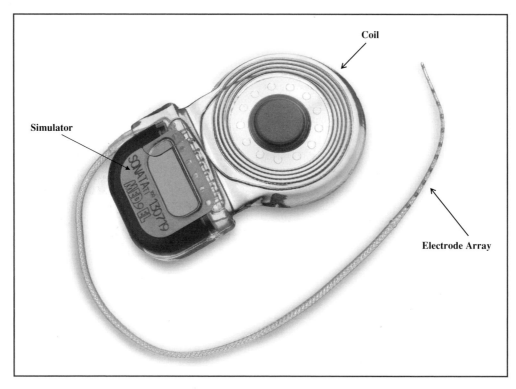

FIGURE 1–14. MED-EL Sonata$_{TI}$^{100} internal device. Courtesy of MED-EL Corporation.

In fact, the electronics and electrode arrays associated with the SONATA$_{TI}^{100}$ are still available in the ceramic casing (i.e., PULSAR$_{CI}^{100}$), which is slightly smaller than the titanium case. Although the titanium casing may improve durability and reduce the chance of failure due to impact trauma, the primary reason MED-EL introduced the titanium casing was to answer surgeons' requests. MED-EL's reliability data have yet to show differences relative to the ceramic casing, which had a relatively low rate of case fracture. The characteristics of the SONATA$_{TI}^{100}$ are provided in Table 1–4. It features a sophisticated digital signal processor with a powerful microchip and several electrode array options. The SONATA$_{TI}^{100}$ also offers a two-way telemetry system for transmission of the signal to the internal device and acquisition of information from the internal device.

The digital signal processor allows for a total maximum stimulation rate of 50,704 pulses per second. It has independent output circuits for each channel, enabling precise delivery of stimulation and providing the future capability for simultaneous activation of channels. Twenty-four oval electrode contacts are arranged in pairs to form 12 stimulating sites. The paired configuration allows for a broader stimulation site and allows the same electrode array to be used for either the right or left ear. A primary return (or reference) electrode and a secondary reference electrode (i.e., EAP) are located on the titanium casing. (For the PULSAR$_{CI}^{100}$ the reference electrode is a remote lead positioned under the temporalis muscle.) The EAP reference electrode is used for recording the electrically evoked compound action potential via Auditory nerve Response Telemetry (ART).

One unique and potentially beneficial aspect of the standard MED-EL electrode array is the 31.5 mm array length from the apical end to the seal placed in the cochleostomy. Electrode arrays offered by other manufacturers typically extend about 25 mm into the cochlea. Deeper insertion of the electrode array may provide better access to low-frequency sounds because stimulation will be provided to the region most sensitive and tonotopically organized to low frequencies (rather than providing low-frequency sounds in the region of the auditory system sensitive to mid frequencies).

Also, it allows for greater spacing between electrode contact pairs, potentially reducing channel interaction. The three special array options include the Medium Electrode Array (HM), the Split Electrode Array (HGB), and the Compressed Electrode Array (HS). The Standard Array electrode contacts are arranged 26.4 mm across the array with 2.4 mm between each contact pair. This design allows for stimulation in the most apical regions of the cochlea and some distance between stimulating contacts. This array is recommended for most recipients. The Medium Array electrode contacts span 20.9 mm across the array with a 1.9 mm space between each stimulating site. This array may be used when a deep insertion is not possible (e.g., abnormal cochlear anatomy or reimplantation after previous use of another brand). Finally, the Compressed Array electrode contacts are placed 12.1 mm across the array with 1.1 mm spacing between sites. This array is intended for recipients who have ossification or fibrous tissue growth in the cochlea. The Split Array is used for cases in which significant ossification exists in the cochlea. The 12 contact pairs are arranged on 2 separate electrode arrays that use the same spacing as the compressed array; 7 channels are on one array and 5 channels are on the other. When using this array, the surgeon must make two cochleostomy sites to insert one array into the upper-basal turn of the cochlea and the other into the lower-basal region. Likewise, the audiologist must reorder the tonotopic arrangement of the bandpass filters at the initial programming, depending on which of the two electrode arrays was placed in the lower basal turn and which was place in the upper turn of the cochlea.

KEY CONCEPTS

Following this chapter, the reader should recognize and understand the following concepts:

- The basic operation of cochlear implants is similar across the three manufacturers.
- The basic components of cochlear implant systems also are similar across manufacturers.

■ The internal devices and sound processors across manufacturers each have several distinctive characteristics, programming parameters, and user controls.

║║║ 2 ║║║

Basic Terminology of Cochlear Implant Programming

Although several parallels exist between cochlear implants and hearing aids, numerous differences occur in the terminology used in the programming of each device. The goal of this chapter is to familiarize the reader with fundamental terms and concepts that are encountered when programming a cochlear implant. The first half of the chapter discusses how three sets of parameters influence the acoustical components of the signal in the following domains: (1) intensity, (2) frequency, and (3) time. The second half of the chapter addresses basic terminology associated with contemporary cochlear implants and signal coding strategies.

PARAMETERS AFFECTING SIGNAL CODING IN THE INTENSITY DOMAIN

A summary of the parameters that influence coding in the intensity domain are provided in Table 2–1.

Stimulation Levels

One of the most important parameters a clinician determines when programming a recipient's cochlear implant is the magnitude of stimulation provided from the implant to the auditory nerve. The fundamental goal of programming is to restore audibility for a range of speech sounds extending from soft speech to loud speech. Ideally, stimulation levels also are set to optimize identification of speech sounds. Finally, it is desirable to set stimulation levels so that normal loudness percepts are restored for speech in addition to environmental sounds. Sounds that are perceived as soft to a person with normal-hearing sensitivity also should sound soft to a cochlear implant user, while sounds that are perceived as loud for a person with normal-hearing sensitivity also should be loud, but not uncomfortable to the user.

Achieving the aforementioned goals is challenging because speech and everyday acoustical sounds have a wide range of intensities of approximately 100 dB. For most cochlear implant users, this wide range of intensities must be coded into a relatively small electrical dynamic range (often around 20 dB when converted from clinical units to dB; Nelson, Schmitz, Donaldson, Viemeister, & Javel, 1996; Zeng & Galvin, 1999). The electrical dynamic range is defined as the difference between the cochlear implant user's perceptual threshold and most comfortable level (i.e., loud but not uncomfortable) for electrical stimulation. Cochlear implant manufacturers use various types of compression to code the acoustic inputs of interest

Table 2–1. Summary of Factors Affecting Signal Coding in the Intensity Domain

Term	Description
Threshold (T level, THR)	Softest electrical input level detectable by user for each electrode contact
Upper stimulation Level (C level, M level, MCL)	Electrical input level that is perceived as loud, but comfortable to user
Amplitude	Current amplitude per phase of a biphasic electrical pulse
Pulse width	Duration or length of one single phase (typically in microseconds)
Electrical dynamic range	Difference in electrical units between threshold and upper stimulation level
Input dynamic range (IDR)	Range of acoustic inputs mapped into electrical dynamic range
Sensitivity	Determines gain of processor microphone, which subsequently determines the quietest sound picked up by the microphone
Channel gain	Controls per-channel location of stimulation within the electrical dynamic range
Volume	Determines the upper stimulation level setting used by the recipient, which subsequently determines the loudness level of the incoming acoustic signal

into the recipient's measured electrical dynamic range. This section introduces programming parameters related to the electrical dynamic range, while the following section discusses how these parameters dictate the electrical dynamic range.

Threshold of Stimulation

The threshold of electrical stimulation refers to the least amount of stimulation a recipient can detect when electrical signals (typically biphasic electrical pulses) are delivered to individual electrode contacts. The exact definition and name of the electrical threshold of stimulation varies across programming software manufacturers. For Advanced Bionics cochlear implants, the electrical threshold is comparable to the audiometric threshold and is best defined as the lowest amount of electrical stimulation a user can detect with 50% accuracy. For Cochlear Corporation implants, the electrical threshold is defined as the minimum amount of electrical stimulation the recipient can detect 100% of the time. In contrast, MED-EL defines electrical threshold as the highest level at which a response is not obtained. Abbreviated

terms, such as "T level" for Advanced Bionics and Cochlear Corporation and "THR" or "threshold" level in MED-EL devices, often are used to describe the electrical threshold.

In adults and older children, the measurement of electrical threshold is relatively straightforward and involves psychophysical measures frequently used in diagnostic audiology. Most commonly, recipients are instructed to raise their hands or say "yes" when they hear the pulsed programming signal. To a cochlear implant user, this signal is perceptually similar to a beep or tone used in pure tone audiometric assessment. The clinician usually employs a modified Hughson-Westlake ascending/descending adaptive procedure to determine threshold (Carhart & Jerger, 1959). The ideal step size for testing likely varies by manufacturer because stimulation scales are different. Larger step sizes may be used for young children who have limited attention spans. For some recipients with tinnitus, determination of threshold may be difficult because the signal tends to "blend" with the ongoing tinnitus. This problem is especially prevalent in newly implanted users.

An alternative approach to the measurement of electrical threshold is to ask recipients to count the number of beeps they hear. When using the procedure, the clinician randomly alters the number of signals presented at each trial (typically between two to five beeps at a time), and the user's task is to report accurately the number of beeps heard. This method assists recipients in focusing on a pulsed signal rather than the continuous tinnitus and enhances their likelihood of responding to the signal rather than the tinnitus. Use of a count-the-beeps approach often results in higher thresholds than thresholds based on conventional audiometric threshold procedures (Skinner, Holden, Holden, & Demorest, 1995). According to research, a higher threshold level may improve the salience of soft speech and environmental sounds (Skinner, Holden, Holden, & Demorest, 1999).

Psychophysical loudness scaling is an alternative approach to set the threshold of electrical stimulation. With this method, the clinician typically begins presentation of the signal at a subthreshold level and gradually increases the presentation level over time (i.e., ascending approach). Recipients are asked to acknowledge their loudness percept of the signal by pointing to categories on a loudness scale similar to the scale pictured in Figure 2–1. Electrical threshold typically is set at a level that corresponds to "barely audible" or "very soft" on the scale. Similar to the count-the-beeps approach, this method likely results in higher threshold levels than what is obtained with conventional audiometric procedures. In addition, it results in better detection for low-level speech and environmental sounds (Skinner, Holden, Holden, & Demorest, 1999).

Obtaining threshold levels may be difficult in young children with cochlear implants. The techniques for establishing threshold levels vary by age and are similar to behavioral testing approaches used by pediatric audiologists to evaluate hearing sensitivity. A detailed discussion on the measurement of thresholds in children is provided in Chapter 3.

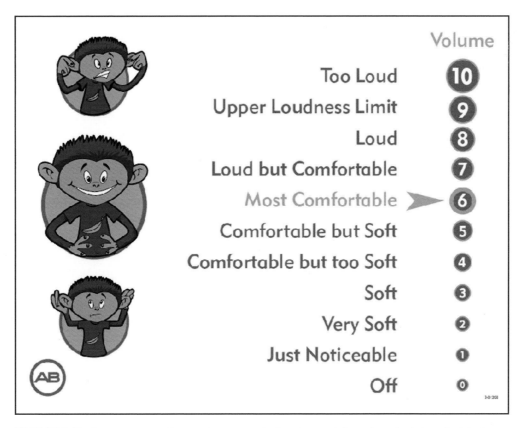

FIGURE 2–1. Example of a loudness scale for determining electrical threshold. Courtesy of Advanced Bionics (http://www.AdvancedBionics.com).

In an effort to expedite the programming process and eliminate an audible noise that may occur when T levels are set too high in CIS-type signal coding strategies, Advanced Bionics and MED-EL introduced programming strategies that do not require the measurement of electrical threshold. Instead, the electrical threshold is set at 0 units of stimulation or a certain percentage (e.g., 10%) of the maximum stimulation level. The magnitude of stimulation provided for low-level inputs is determined by compression processing and logarithmic mapping functions, which place the acoustic input range into the upper portion of the typical recipient's electrical dynamic range. Previous research suggests that speech recognition and audibility for soft sounds are similar when using maps with measured threshold levels versus estimated threshold levels (Spahr & Dorman, 2005). In contrast, Baudhuin, Cadieux, Reeder, Kettel, and Firszt (2009) showed that detection thresholds, for warble-tone stimuli presented in the sounds field, were lower when subjects used programs with measured threshold levels. As a result, in some cases it may be beneficial to measure electrical-threshold levels in programs that use estimated threshold levels as the default, particularly for children who require the audibility of low-level speech sounds for speech recognition and speech and language development. At the very least, clinicians should evaluate a recipients' ability to hear low-level sounds in the soundfield. The audiologist should consider increasing the electrical threshold when behavioral hearing thresholds exceed 30 dB HL for adults or 25 dB HL for children (or adjust other manufacturer-specific parameters that enhance audibility for low-level inputs; in particular, MED-EL recommends adjusting other parameters to improve audibility for low-level sounds). See Chapter 4.

Upper Stimulation Levels

The programming parameter related to the upper level of stimulation varies by terminology and definition across manufacturers. In the Advanced Bionics system, the upper limit of electrical stimulation is set at a level the user perceives as "most comfortable." This parameter is similar to the most comfortable listening level frequently measured in hearing aid evaluations and, in Advanced Bionics cochlear implants, is commonly known as the "M level." In the MED-EL system, upper stimulation levels are known as "maximum comfort levels" (i.e., MCL) and are defined as the amount of electrical stimulation considered to be "loud, but not uncomfortable." For Cochlear Corporation implants, upper stimulation levels are known as C levels and are set to a level of stimulation the user considers to be "loud, but comfortable."

A cochlear implant user's upper stimulation levels are critically important because they influence speech recognition, sound quality, and in the case of prelingually deafened children, the ability to monitor one's own voice and produce intelligible speech. Several users of cochlear implants experience poor outcomes that may be attributed to inappropriate upper stimulation levels. Clinicians typically set upper stimulation levels via psychophysical loudness scaling methods or through behavioral observation. Several researchers report that the electrically evoked stapedial reflex threshold (ESRT) serves as a useful guide for determining upper stimulation levels (Brickley et al., 2005; Buckler & Overstreet, 2003; Wolfe & Kasulis, 2008). A detailed discussion of setting upper stimulation levels is provided in Chapter 3.

Current Amplitude and Pulse Width

As previously mentioned, contemporary cochlear implants deliver biphasic electrical pulses (Figure 2–2) to electrode contacts across the electrode array. Increases in the stimulus intensity can be obtained in two ways. First, the amplitude of the current can be increased. Figure 2–3 provides an example in which the intensity of the original stimulus (2–3a) has been doubled by increasing the current amplitude by a factor of two (2–3b). Second, the stimulus intensity can be increased by lengthening the pulse width. Figure 2–3c illustrates a situation in which the stimulus intensity

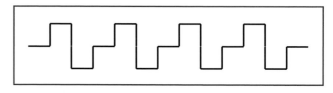

FIGURE 2–2. Illustration of a biphasic electrical pulse.

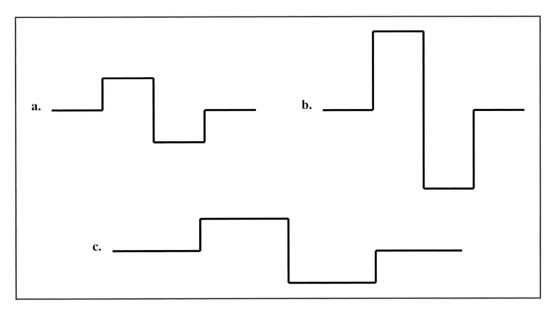

FIGURE 2–3. Increase in intensity from an original signal (**a**) achieved with increased current amplitude (**b**) and increased pulse width (**c**).

has been doubled by increasing the pulse width by a factor of two. Therefore, the total magnitude of a biphasic, electrical pulse is determined by the amplitude of the current and the width of each pulse. The total energy in the stimulus is specified in charge units (Current amplitude * Pulse width = Total charge in nanocoulombs [unit of charge]).

Mapping Acoustical Inputs into the Electrical Dynamic Range

The three cochlear implant manufacturers in the United States take different approaches to directing desirable acoustic inputs into the recipient's electrical dynamic range. The following parameters influence the provision of acoustical inputs into the recipient's electrical dynamic range: input dynamic range, sensitivity, compression, channel gain, and volume control. All of these parameters, as described here, influence the way the signal is coded in the intensity domain. A more detailed explanation of how these parameters are used during programming is provided in Chapter 4.

Input Dynamic Range (IDR)

The input dynamic range of a sound processor is a clinician-adjustable parameter that, along with microphone sensitivity, determines the range of acoustic inputs that are mapped into the recipient's electrical dynamic range. As shown in Figure 2–4, the default IDR of contemporary cochlear implant systems ranges from 40 to 75 dB. The lower end of the IDR determines the acoustic input level that is mapped near the threshold of electrical stimulation, while the upper end of the IDR determines the acoustic input level that is mapped near the maximum electrical stimulation level (i.e., M level, MCL, or C level).

In current cochlear implants, the lower end of the IDR usually is set between 20 to 30 dB SPL, while the upper end of the IDR is set between 65 and 85 dB SPL depending on the manufacturer. Acoustic inputs that fall below the lower end of the IDR are mapped below the recipient's electrical dynamic range and are presumably inaudible to the user. Acoustic inputs that exceed the IDR are subjected to infinite compression. Cochlear Corporation also uses a parameter known as *instantaneous input dynamic range* (IIDR), which refers to the range of short-term fluctuations that are mapped without compression (or other types of attenuation, such as autosensitivity) into the recipient's electrical dynamic range. The IIDR is typically set to 30 to 40 dB SPL in order to capture the range of ongoing speech amplitudes, from peaks to valleys, at a given input level. Cochlear

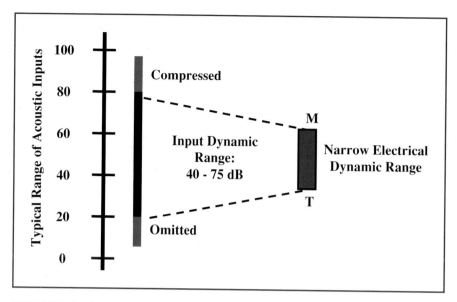

FIGURE 2–4. Illustration of electrical dynamic range as measured in the soundfield and input dynamic range (IDR) in dB SPL. T/THR = threshold; C/M/MCL = most comfortable level.

Corporation defines IDR as the total range of input levels the processor can analyze without clipping or significant distortion. With a change in the sensitivity parameter (either manually or adaptively via signal processing within the sound processor), a wider range of acoustic inputs is delivered to the recipient's electrical dynamic range as overall input levels change.

Sensitivity

The parameter known as sensitivity controls the gain provided by the sound processor microphone. For Cochlear Corporation implants, sensitivity is also referred to as microphone sensitivity. The numerical value of the sensitivity parameter varies by manufacturer and is discussed more thoroughly in Chapter 4.

Sensitivity interacts with the IDR/IIDR parameter to determine how acoustic inputs are mapped into the recipient's electrical dynamic range. In essence, a reduction in microphone sensitivity adjusts the IDR in a predictable manner. As shown in Figure 2–5 when the microphone sensitivity is reduced from a default setting of 12 to a lower setting (e.g., closer to zero), the acoustic input level required to engage the high-level

compressor increases. Also, the floor of the IDR/IIDR increases to reduce the audibility of low-level sounds. Conversely, if the microphone sensitivity is increased above the default setting, audibility for low-level sounds is improved and acoustic inputs below the default ceiling of the IDR/IIDR are subjected to infinite compression. Overall, the sensitivity control makes adjustments to the input signal prior to frequency analysis; therefore, its effect is similar across the frequency range of the processor.

Compression

All contemporary cochlear implant systems use compression to direct a wide range of acoustic inputs into the implant user's narrow electrical dynamic range. In essence, the compression acts as an automatic gain control, but the gain adjustment as a function of input level varies widely across manufacturers. For example, all three U.S. commercial cochlear implant systems use a feature known as Automatic Gain Control (AGC), but the manner in which this feature is implemented is very different among the three systems. Certain characteristics of the AGC in the Advanced Bionics and MED-EL systems can be adjusted by

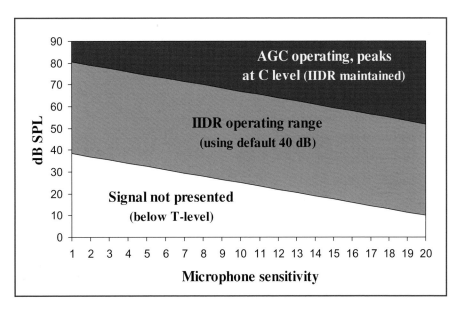

FIGURE 2–5. Relationship of microphone sensitivity setting to compression and audibility of high- and low-level sounds. Courtesy of Cochlear™ Americas, © 2005 Cochlear Ltd.

the clinician (see Chapter 4). However, Cochlear Corporation systems offers a special type of input processing known as *autosensitivity*, which basically operates like a slow-acting compressor in response to moderate- to high-level input noise.

Channel Gain

Adjustments to channel gain controls the amplification provided to the signal in a channel-specific and, therefore, frequency-specific manner. Similar to the other parameters, the effect of changing the channel gain varies by manufacturer. In cochlear implant systems using CIS-type strategies, an increase of the channel gain results in a frequency-specific increase to the input signal. An increase in channel gain should enhance the salience of the signal in a frequency-specific manner without the need for increases in the upper stimulation level. This may be appealing when increases in the upper stimulation level produce undesirable effects, such as poor sound quality, facial nerve stimulation, discomfort, etc.

For the Cochlear Corporation device, adjustment of the channel gain also affects the signal in a frequency-specific manner as it leaves the sound processor microphone. In other words, the effect

of gain occurs prior to the processing of the signal. As a result, the effect of channel gain on the signal varies by the signal coding strategy and may result in certain sounds being more or less likely to be delivered to the electrode contacts for stimulation of the auditory nerve. The effect of channel gain is discussed further in Chapter 4.

Volume Control

In general, the volume control parameter is fairly straightforward. As one would expect, adjustments to the volume control affect the user's perception of signal loudness. For all three systems commercially available in the United States, a change in the volume control setting produces a change in the upper level of stimulation (i.e., C levels, M levels, or MCL). Depending on the programmed settings, however, adjusting the volume control to the minimal position may result in little to no sound percept for the patient, or this action may result in a minimal change in overall stimulation. Furthermore, changing the volume control setting to the maximum position may result in only a small change to stimulation levels, or this action may result in a dramatic increase in the upper stimulation level. Therefore, it is very important that the clinician and patient share a thorough understanding of the effect of the volume control on the stimulation provided to the user.

PARAMETERS AFFECTING SIGNAL CODING IN THE FREQUENCY DOMAIN

Electrode Contact versus Channel

As described in Chapter 1, the term *electrode contact* describes a physical contact in the internal device electrode array where stimulation is delivered to the auditory nerve fibers. The term *intracochlear electrode contact* describes an electrode contact located inside the cochlea and used for the delivery of stimulation to auditory nerve fibers. The number of intracochlear electrode contacts varies across manufacturers (Advanced Bionics: 16, Cochlear Corporation: 22, and MED-EL: 24 electrode contacts arranged in pairs to create 12 separate stimulation sites). Frequency information in the incoming acoustic signal is primarily conveyed by the place of stimulation within the cochlea. Cochlear implant signal coding strategies take advantage of the tonotopic organization of the typically functioning cochlea by delivering low-frequency inputs to electrode contacts located in the apical end of the cochlea and high-frequency inputs to electrode contacts located in the basal end of the cochlea.

A *channel* describes a discrete frequency range over which sound is analyzed for eventual delivery to an electrode contact. Channels are defined by bandpass filters with a relatively steep roll-off (although overlap may exist between neighboring channels). In many cases, electrode contacts and stimulation are similar. For instance, as seen in Figure 2–6, inputs that are processed through channel 1 are delivered to electrode contact number 1. In other cases, the channel number and electrode number may be different. As seen in Figure 2–7, inputs processed through channel 1 are actually delivered to electrode 2, and inputs processed through channel 2 are delivered to electrode 1. In the latter case, adjustments were made to improve the patient's tonotopic organization. The subject's pitch percept did not transition in the expected low-to-high manner when stimulation was swept across the electrodes. Therefore, switching the channel to electrode assignment restored the desired tonotopic organization. Double channel mapping is another example in which the inputs from two channels are delivered to one electrode, but this topic will be discussed in greater detail in Chapter 4.

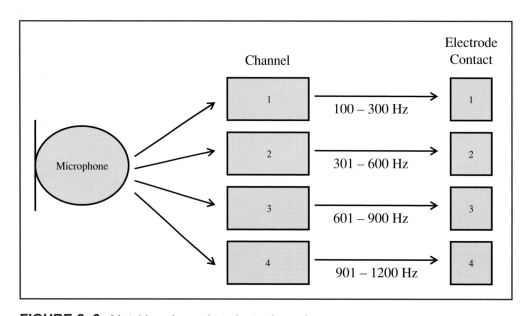

FIGURE 2–6. Matching channel to electrode assignment.

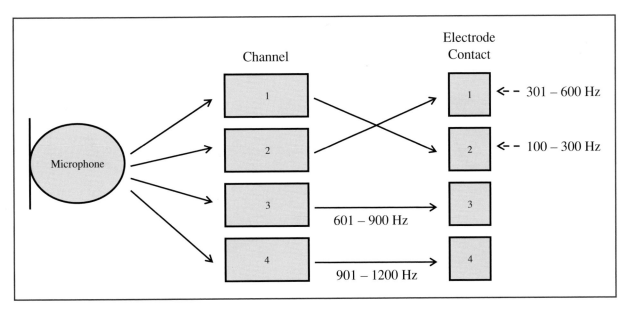

FIGURE 2–7. Switching channel to electrode assignment to restore tonotopicity.

Virtual Electrodes (Current Steering)

Advanced Bionics and MED-EL use a relatively new concept (in clinical implementation) known as virtual electrodes or current steering. In the Advanced Bionics current-steering approach, two neighboring electrodes are stimulated simultaneously, resulting in a focal provision of stimulation between the two contacts. As seen in Figure 2–8a, when two neighboring electrodes are stimulated simultaneously with equal magnitude, the focus of stimulation falls within the middle of the two electrodes. If the magnitude of stimulation is greater at one of the electrodes, then the focus of stimulation will occur closer to that electrode (Figure 2–8b).

Intermediate pitches also can be created using sequential stimulation, as implemented in the current MED-EL approach, and require the use of bell-shaped overlapping bandpass filters to elicit pitch percepts that shift gradually within and across channels along the electrode array. The Cochlear Nucleus implant also has the capability of applying current steering through sequential stimulation, but at this point, the approach is not used in clinically available signal coding strategies.

The objective of this approach is to increase the spectral-resolution abilities of recipients. The normal cochlea contains about 3,500 inner hair cells, each of which is tonotopically tuned to one individual frequency and one corresponding afferent auditory nerve fiber. This exquisite design of the normal peripheral auditory system allows for discrimination between acoustic components that differ by approximately 2 Hz (Wier, Jesteadt, & Green, 1977). Adept spectral resolution is critical for discrimination of consonants that differ on the basis of place cues, optimal recognition of melodies and enjoyment of music, and speech recognition in the presence of competing noise. Given the fact that cochlear implants provide far fewer transduction sites than the normal ear (12 to 22 physical electrode contacts versus 3,500 inner hair cells), the concept of virtual electrodes (current steering) is an attempt to increase the spectral fidelity of the signal delivered to the auditory nerve. The clinical implementation of this concept along with expected clinical benefit is discussed in Chapter 4.

Frequency Allocation

As the name implies, the parameter frequency allocation controls how frequencies are delivered across the active channels. In the Advanced Bionics

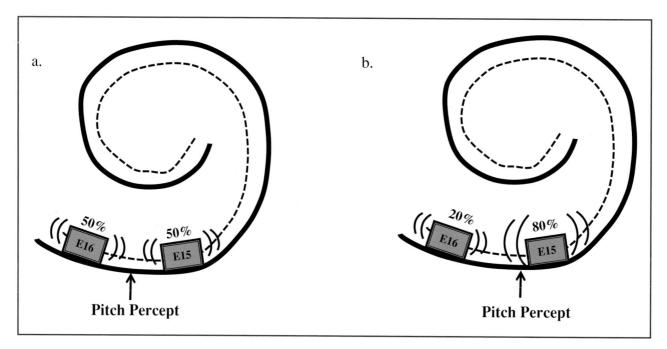

FIGURE 2–8. Illustration of current steering. (**a**) Two neighboring electrodes stimulated simultaneously with equal magnitude; (**b**) two neighboring electrodes stimulated simultaneously, but one with greater magnitude.

system, frequency allocation is determined automatically by the programming software. If an electrode is disabled, the frequencies then are reallocated to existing active electrodes. In the Cochlear Corporation devices, adjustment of the frequency allocation parameter affects the higher limit (or the highest frequency to be delivered to the most basal electrode), as well as the width of bandpass filters in the midfrequency channels. An additional parameter in the Cochlear Corporation programming software referred to as " edit frequency boundaries," allows the clinician to specify the exact cut-off frequencies of each channel. In the MED-EL device, clinicians may change the lower (70 to 350 Hz) and higher (3,500 to 8,500 Hz) frequency limits in 10- and 500-Hz intervals, respectively. Also, clinicians can select from four different frequency allocation tables that are each based on different psychoacoustically derived approaches. Additional information on the frequency allocation for the Cochlear Corporation and MED-EL devices is provided in Chapter 4.

PARAMETERS AFFECTING SIGNAL CODING IN THE TIME DOMAIN

Stimulation Rate

As stated previously, contemporary cochlear implant systems deliver trains of biphasic electrical pulses to the intracochlear electrode contacts. The stimulation rate typically refers to the number of biphasic pulses that are delivered to an individual electrode contact within one second and is specified in pulses per second (pps). The earliest multiple channel cochlear implants had relatively slow stimulation rates (i.e., 250 pps or less), but contemporary systems allow for much higher stimulation rates (i.e., up to about 5,000 pps). Aside from coding temporal cues, changes in stimulation rate also can result in changes in the user's pitch and intensity percepts. Specifically, faster stimulation rates often result in a louder signal due to temporal summation and a higher pitch percept, particularly as rate is increased from 50 to 500 Hz.

Theoretical benefits can be gained by providing higher rates of stimulation. First, the incoming acoustic signals change in amplitude over time. Slow changes in amplitude (i.e., 2 to 50 Hz) provide the user with an amplitude envelope. The envelope provides temporal cues used to understand speech. Conversely, rapid fluctuations in amplitude carry information about the fine temporal structure of the signal. Acquisition of fine temporal structure is critical for speech understanding in noise, music recognition and appreciation, and potentially, recognition of vocal pitch. Finally, the amplitude envelope and spectrum of some speech sounds are similar; therefore, the listener must rely on differences in fine temporal structure to discern among sounds.

Additionally, stimulation of the auditory nerve with electrical pulses results in a highly synchronous compound response from auditory nerve fibers adjacent to the electrode contact. The normal auditory system, however, responds in a stochastic manner to acoustic stimulation. A stochastic response occurs when some auditory nerve fibers are excited in response to an individual acoustic stimulus while others are not because they are in their refractory or recovery period.

Another important concept related to stimulation rate is the refractoriness of the auditory nerve fibers. The normal auditory system is capable of following changes in amplitude of an acoustic signal in a time-locked manner (Moller, 2001, 2006; Moore, 2003). This property of the normal auditory system may be beneficial because it theoretically allows the system to follow high-frequency stimuli in a per-cycle manner and provides for the acquisition of fine temporal structure. Moller (2001, 2006) also contends that the temporal response of the auditory nerve plays a critical role in the processing of pitch and frequency. He notes that an auditory nerve fiber cannot respond to each individual cycle of a stimulus because some fibers are still in a refractory state. Fibers likely respond to multiples of the incoming stimulus rate. However, the auditory nerve fibers collectively are able to follow the stimulus on a cycle-by-cycle rate.

This phenomenon has previously been referred to as the "volley approach."

When using electrical stimulation rates below 2,000 pps, the auditory nerve fires in a highly synchronous manner. Because the auditory nerve fibers are firing in unison, and subsequently possess a simultaneous refractory period, the auditory system is unable to follow rapid changes in a stimulus (i.e., fine temporal structure). At stimulation rates above 2,000 pps, the auditory nerve is more likely to assume stochastic firing, and as a result, a higher probability exists that the nerve fibers will respond in a volley type fashion to follow fine temporal structure cues.

In reality, a paucity of research demonstrates consistent improvements in patient performance when stimulation rates exceed 2,000 pps. According to research, subjects who converted from slower (800–1,600 pps) to faster (5,000 pps) coding strategies achieved better speech recognition (Dunn, Tyler, Witt, & Gantz, 2006; Koch, Osberger, Segel, & Kessler, 2004). However, the subjects in the Koch et al. study had a longer duration of experience with the higher rate coding strategy; therefore, the improvement may be attributed to learning effects. Also, in both studies, the faster strategy provided twice as many stimulation sites (i.e., electrode contacts) and had a more sophisticated AGC. As a result, other signal processing variables may have been responsible for performance gains.

Most researchers who are exploring performance changes as a function of stimulation rate conclude that the optimal stimulation rate varies on an individual basis (Arora, Dawson, Dowell, & Vandali, 2009; Balkany et al., 2007; Buchner, Frohne-Buchner, Battmer, & Lenarz 2004; Vandali, Whitford, Plant, & Clark, 2000). Clearly, stimulation rates up to several hundred pulses per second seem to be beneficial for all cochlear implant users. Some recipients, however, achieve maximum performance and prefer rates of 500 pps, and others prefer and perform optimally with rates of up to 5,000 pps (Buchner et al.). As a result, the user probably is best served by a clinician who identifies the individual's optimal stimulation rate.

The optimal stimulation rate may vary on the basis of cochlear implant hardware as well. To optimize the delivery of high-rate electrical pulses, the current sources of the implant's internal device must be able to generate narrow pulse widths with high current amplitudes. Also, the spacing between electrode contacts may influence a recipient's performance with higher stimulation rates as closer spacing may increase the likelihood of temporal channel interaction. Indeed, reduced channel interaction seems to play a role in better performance with high-rate stimuli as some studies have shown that performance with very fast stimulation rates (e.g., 5,000 pps) is more likely with 8-channel maps (every other electrode contact disabled) versus 16-channel programs in which all active electrode contacts are enabled (Buchner et al., 2004). Furthermore, the sampling rate of the sound processor must be fast enough to capture the fast fluctuations occurring in the input signal (i.e., the sampling rate must be at least twice as high as the highest frequency of interest in the incoming sound). More research is needed to explore the potential benefits and limitations of high stimulation rates across the variety of cochlear implant systems available on the commercial market. The optimal stimulation rate may vary across users and device characteristics.

Manufacturers also frequently refer to a total stimulation rate, or the overall maximum rate of stimulation possible, across all active electrodes within one second. Total stimulation rate usually is calculated by determining the product of the per channel stimulation rate and the number of active channels stimulated for an incoming stimulus (per channel stimulation rate * number of active channels stimulated = total stimulation rate). For example, if an incoming sound is delivered to 10 channels, and the per channel stimulation rate is 1,200 pps, the total stimulation rate is 12,000 pps.

The maximum total stimulation rate usually is determined by the number of pulses per second the implant is capable of delivering. There are, however, exceptions to this rule. For instance, the Cochlear Corporation CI512 device is capable of a total stimulation rate of 32,000 pps. However, when the ACE signal coding strategy is selected, the total stimulation rate is 14,400 pps. This limited total stimulation rate for ACE is historically based. When ACE was developed for commercial use, the Nucleus 24 implant was the internal device available at the time, and it was capable

of a total stimulation rate of only 14,400 pps. To access higher total stimulation rates in the Nucleus CI512 device, the clinician must select the more recently developed "High-ACE" (ACE-RE) coding strategy.

BASIC COCHLEAR IMPLANT TERMINOLOGY

Basic definitions for cochlear implant programming terminology are provided in Table 2–2.

Electrode Coupling Strategy/ Stimulation Mode

The electrode coupling strategy (or stimulation mode) indicates how channels are connected to form an electrical circuit through which current can be delivered to the auditory nerve. In a complete electrical circuit, current travels from the power source to a resistive component and then to a return location. Cochlear implant stimulation must also be delivered through a complete circuit.

The "electrical circuit" in a cochlear implant is made up of (1) the signal generator in the internal processor (current source/output circuit), (2) the active electrode lead and contact, and (3) return electrode(s). Depending upon the application, the clinician's preferred terminology, and the manufacturer, the return electrodes also may be referred to as ground, indifferent, or reference electrodes. The electrode contact, cochlear fluids, and other tissues adjacent to the active electrode contact serve as the resistive elements in this circuit. The active electrode is always an intracochlear electrode and ideally is located in the scala tympani. In contemporary cochlear implants, the return electrode(s) usually is an extracochlear electrode (located outside of the cochlea). The return electrode typically is located on the case of the internal stimulator. Alternatively, it may be located on the electrode lead or within a separate lead that terminates in a electrode contact at a remote location from the cochlea (see Chapter 1).

Monopolar stimulation describes electrode coupling in which stimulation is provided to an

Table 2–2. Summary of Basic Cochlear Implant Programming Terminology

Term	Description
Electrode Coupling Strategy/Stimulation Mode	How electrodes are electrically connected to form an electrical circuit; all consist of active and reference electrodes
Sequential Stimulation	Presentation of biphasic pulses to electrodes occur one after another
Simultaneous & Partially Simultaneous Stimulation	Presentation of biphasic pulses are directed to several or two (partial) electrodes at one time
Sweeping	Sequential presentation of a programming stimulus across the electrode array (typically at C/M/MCL level to ensure user comfort)
Loudness Balancing	Successive presentation of stimulus to two or more electrodes; ensures equal loudness
Radio Frequency	The carrier frequency for transmission of signals across scalp: from processor to internal device and/or vice versa
Bidirectional Telemetry	Transmission of signals to and from the implant. Used for normal stimulation, device programming, and to check integrity of internal device
Electrical Impedance	Measurement of electrode function: the amount of current that returns to a reference electrode
Voltage Compliance	Maximum amount of current delivered to electrode for a given power source
Mixing Ratio	Relative strength of signals from processor and auxiliary input source

Note. C/M/MCL = most comfortable level of electrical stimulation for given electrode.

active intracochlear electrode and an extracochlear electrode serves as the return (Figure 2–9). All contemporary cochlear implants use monopolar stimulation as the default mode. An alternative approach is *bipolar stimulation*, that is bipolar electrode coupling whereby electrical current is delivered to an active intracochlear electrode and a neighboring intracochlear electrode serves as the return (Figure 2–10). Bipolar coupling specifically is referred to as bipolar stimulation (BP) when the return electrode is positioned immediately adjacent to the active electrode. When the return and active electrodes are separated by one electrode contact, the bipolar stimulation is referred to as bipolar +1 (BP+1). BP+2 refers to two electrode contacts separating the active and return electrodes; BP+3 refers to three electrode contacts separating the active and return electrodes; and so forth.

Although bipolar stimulation should provide more focused stimulation, monopolar stimulation does allow for the provision of a tonotopic signal across the cochlea. Additionally, the rela-

tively narrow spread of electrical current inherent with bipolar stimulation requires higher current levels (i.e., higher threshold and upper stimulation levels) to reach a given sound percept when compared to monopolar stimulation. Thus, the higher current levels required for bipolar stimulation may reduce battery life. Furthermore, the broader stimulation pattern provided by monopolar stimulation results in a relatively gradual change in stimulation levels (i.e., T levels and C/M/MCL levels), so interpolation is a viable option in the monopolar mode (see explanation of interpolation later in this chapter). In contrast, stimulation requirements may change drastically from one electrode to the next with bipolar stimulation; therefore, the clinician must measure T and C/M/MCL levels for all active electrodes.

Common ground coupling is another electrode coupling mode used for diagnostic purposes but typically is not used for signal coding. In common ground coupling, electrical current is delivered to an active intracochlear electrode, and all

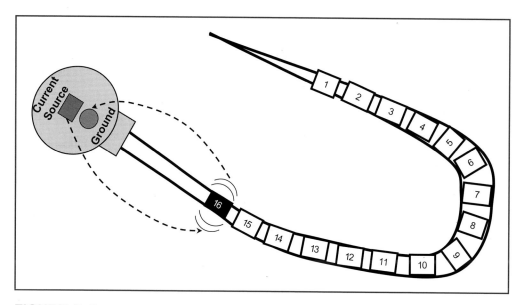

FIGURE 2–9. Illustration of monopolar electrode coupling in which the single reference/ground electrode is at a distance from the active electrodes.

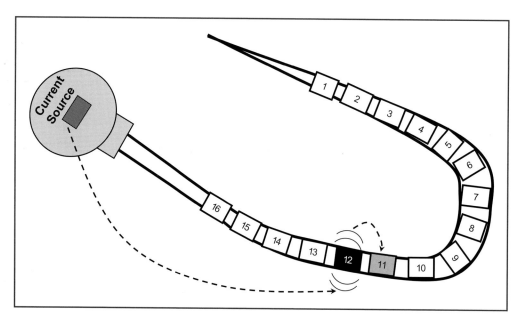

FIGURE 2–10. Illustration of bipolar electrode coupling in which the reference/ground electrode is in close proximity to the active electrode.

of the remaining intracochlear electrodes serve as the collective return (Figure 2–11). Because all of the electrodes are coupled to one another electrically and electrical resistance across these electrodes can be referenced to an extracochlear electrode serving as the ground (defined as zero voltage potential/ reference potential), common ground coupling is the most sensitive mode to detect shorted electrodes during electrode impedance assessment.

Finally, the cochlear implant manufacturers are exploring more advanced electrode coupling strategies, such as tripolar coupling and other higher

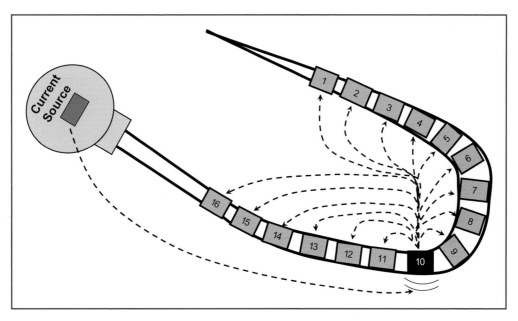

FIGURE 2–11. Illustration of common ground coupling in which all electrodes adjacent to the active electrode serve as the reference/ground electrode.

order coupling modes. The potential advantage of higher order coupling modes is to provide more focused stimulation to spiral ganglion dendrites and cell bodies. At the time of this writing, however, no commercial cochlear implant systems allow for these advanced methods of electrode coupling.

Sequential versus Simultaneous Stimulation

Most contemporary cochlear implant systems deliver electrical biphasic pulses in a sequential fashion, in which the presentation of pulses occurs one after another. In other words, a simultaneous presentation of two pulses never occurs. This approach is designed to reduce or prevent channel interaction, which may result in distortion or smearing of speech sounds. The previously mentioned concept of virtual channels is a variation of simultaneous stimulation that is intended to elicit one percept or "channel" of stimulation. This approach differs from the traditional concept of simultaneous stimulation, which sought to stimulate across several channels at one time.

In contrast to sequential stimulation, simul-taneous stimulation refers to the presentation of an electrical signal to several electrodes at one time. An early signal coding strategy called Simultaneous Analog Stimulation (SAS) used simultaneous stimulation. Zwolan et al. (2001) showed that Advanced Bionics users with low stimulation level needs (i.e., low T and M levels) frequently performed well and preferred the SAS strategy, while recipients with higher stimulation level needs preferred sequential stimulation. Simultaneous stimulation typically is implemented with bipolar electrode coupling in an attempt to reduce channel interaction. Current signal coding strategies do not use totally simultaneous stimulation, primarily to avoid channel interaction.

Advanced Bionics cochlear implants use a combination of the two aforementioned approaches, which may be described as partially simultaneous stimulation. With this approach, biphasic electrical pulses are provided simultaneously to two different electrode contacts, but these electrode contacts are separated by a relatively large physical distance (Figure 2–12). The objective of this approach is to allow for faster rates of stimulation while limiting channel interaction historically associated with simultaneous stimulation.

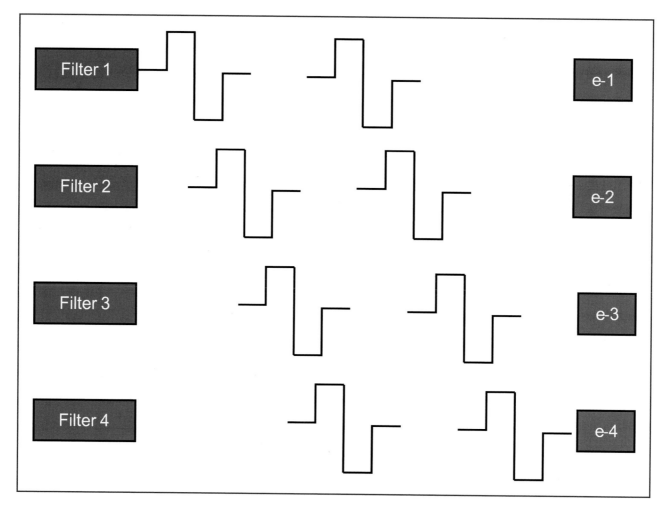

FIGURE 2–12. Illustration of partially simultaneous stimulation.

Interpolation

As the number of cochlear implant recipients has grown, cochlear implant clinicians have struggled to manage their expanding patient caseloads. In response, manufacturers have developed streamlined programming strategies to expedite the programming process. Interpolation refers to the estimation of stimulation levels on the basis of measured values from neighboring channels. For instance, if the measured T levels for electrodes 6 and 8 were 70 and 90, respectively, the estimated T level for electrode 7 would be 80. In practice, interpolation often is used to estimate the stimulation levels for several electrodes that are between two measured electrodes (e.g., electrodes 21–17 are estimated on the basis of measured values at electrodes 22 and 16). Research demonstrates that, on average, user performance for a large group of recipients did not decline when programs were based on interpolated versus individual channel measures (Plant et al., 2005). However, because of individual subject variation, the authors recommend that clinicians measure stimulation levels on most, if not all, active channels when time allows.

Sweeping

Sweeping refers to the sequential presentation of the programming stimulus across the active electrodes at a given stimulation level. Sweeping often is performed at the upper stimulation level (i.e., C/M/MCL level) to ensure that none of the electrodes are too loud or result in unfavorable sound quality. Sweeping, however, may be performed at lower stimulation levels (i.e., 50% of the dynamic range) to ensure equal loudness for lower level inputs, particularly when the recipient complains that certain soft sounds are too loud or that soft speech is difficult to understand. Additionally, the perceived pitch should become progressively higher if sweeping is performed from the apical to basal direction. As such, the prudent clinician may choose to sweep at the upper stimulation level and ensure that the pitch changes in the expected tonotopic manner. Finally, sweeping may be performed across all active electrodes in succession or just across a couple or a few electrodes at a time to allow for more precise responses.

Loudness Balancing

Loudness balancing refers to the successive presentation of a programming stimulus to two or more active electrodes to ensure that the subject perceives the stimuli to be equally loud when each is presented at a specified percentage of the dynamic range. Researchers have reported that the provision of stimulation resulting in equal loudness percepts across the electrode array results in optimal sound quality and speech recognition (Dawson, Skok, & Clark, 1997; Sainz, de la Torre, Roldan, Ruiz, & Vargas, 2003). Most commonly in clinical practice, two or more electrodes are stimulated at the upper stimulation level (i.e., C/M/MCL level), and the subject reports whether the stimuli are equally loud or whether one electrode possesses a louder percept. If the latter is the case, the clinician makes an adjustment to achieve balanced loudness between the electrodes. Typically, the clinician begins with presentation to an active electrode at the most apical location in the electrode array and progresses across electrodes in a basal direction. The number of electrodes that are balanced in a given trial often varies across clinicians (i.e., balancing two, three, four, or more at a time), but the authors prefer to balance loudness across two electrodes. For example, if the clinician begins by asking the recipient to judge loudness at C level for electrodes 22 and 21, and electrode 21 is louder than

22, the stimulation level for electrode 21 should be decreased slightly. The loudness of the two then would be reevaluated. After the recipient reports loudness balance between the electrodes, the clinician compares loudness at C level between electrodes 21 and 20 and eventually for the rest of the electrode array. The adjustment to the stimulation level always should be made to the second electrode in the pair because the first electrode is balanced to the preceding electrodes in the array.

Radio Frequency (RF)

As mentioned in Chapter 1, cochlear implants transmit signals across the scalp via a Radio Frequency (RF) signal. The term RF is frequently used to express the carrier frequency of the radio signal on which the signal of interest is modulated. Some cochlear implant systems use a single RF to transmit signals both to and from the internal device, but the Advanced Bionics Corporation uses one RF for forward transmission and a second RF for backward transmission.

Telemetry

When programming cochlear implants, telemetry refers to the transmission of data through radio-frequency communication to and from the internal implant via the electromagnetic induction link. In other words, telemetry is used to send the signal of interest to the internal device for eventual stimulation. Additionally, telemetry is used during the programming session to deliver signals (i.e., T level stimuli) to the implant. Finally, backward telemetry may be used to transmit signals from the internal device to the external coil, sound processor, and programming computer. Backward telemetry allows the clinician to evaluate the integrity of the internal device and measure responses from the auditory nerve. It also allows for an estimation of the amount of power the internal device needs from the processor.

The term "lock" is often used to specify successful radio communication (i.e., telemetry)

between the internal and external processors. "Failure to obtain lock" happens when the signal cannot be transmitted from the external processor to the internal processor or vice versa.

Electrode Impedance

Electrode impedance is a measure of the opposition to electrical current flow across an electrode to surrounding tissues. This measurement should be conducted at the beginning of every programming session. During the measurement, a small amount of electrical current, which is typically inaudible to the recipient, is delivered sequentially to each active intracochlear electrode. The actual impedance measure result indicates the current that returns to a ground electrode and how voltage is distributed to the stimulated electrode contact (and in some cases, the remaining intracochlear electrode contacts) relative to a ground electrode. Ideally, electrode impedances will be greater than 1 kohm and less than 20 kohms. An electrode with an excessively low impedance (e.g., <1 kohm) is sometimes referred to as a *short*, while an electrode with an excessively high impedance (e.g., >30 kohms) is called an *open circuit*. A short circuit refers to an establishment of relatively low resistance between two points in a circuit, which typically are separated by a much higher electrical resistance. Essentially, the term "short" means that two electrode leads/contacts are electrically coupled to one another. As a result, a shorted electrode is identified as two electrodes that are electrically connected and consequently possess an identical voltage that is distributed to each electrode when only one is stimulated.

Short circuits may be caused by physical contact between two electrode contacts or electrode leads, an electrical fault within the electrode lead/contact, or excessive distortion or tension on the array. Short circuits should be considered as permanent anomalies and remain disabled. Open circuits may be caused by anomalies (e.g., ossification) or by an air bubble or protein buildup in the electrode-tissue interface. These electrodes may assume normal impedance values over time or after a period of electrical stimulation. Furthermore, open circuits may be caused by broken

electrode leads. Electrodes' open circuits should also be disabled but reevaluated after a period of implant use. From a practical standpoint, the most recent version of each manufacturer's software identifies the presence of abnormal electrodes and "flags" them for management by the programming clinician.

Along with the absolute impedance value of each electrode, clinicians also may observe the morphology of electrode impedances (i.e., shape or change of impedances across the electrode array) and changes in impedance values across time. Ideally, electrode impedance values should be relatively similar across the electrode array or vary gradually. Erratic electrode impedance patterns should be evaluated more closely.

It is normal for electrode impedances to be relatively high (e.g., 10 to 20 kohms) at cochlear implant activation because of air bubbles or protein buildup around the electrode contact. These values should decrease within the first few days of implant use and eventually stabilize during the first few weeks of electrical stimulation. If electrode values continue to fluctuate after several months of use, the programming clinician should monitor recipient performance closely and consider a referral to an otologist for medical evaluation. In this case, a representative of the manufacturer also should be notified. Electrode conditioning is a feature available in some implant systems that allows for the presentation of low-level current to each electrode to remove air bubbles, protein buildup, etc. Electrode conditioning is needed only prior to testing in the operating room, at initial activation, or when activating electrodes that were previously disabled. Finally, it is normal for electrode impedance to increase slightly with prolonged periods of nonuse of the implant (e.g., if external equipment is broken for several days). These impedances should resume typical values when the implant use is resumed.

Abnormal electrode impedance values may compromise sound quality or produce nonauditory sensations, such as facial nerve stimulation. Other detrimental effects associated with the use of abnormal electrodes include poor speech-recognition performance, inadequate loudness growth, sudden changes in loudness, and potential discomfort.

Numerous reasons for changes or fluctuations in impedance exist. For instance, the electrode array may become displaced over time. Also, ossification or fibrous tissue may arise in the cochlea after implantation and alter the electrode-neural tissue interface. A Stenver's x-ray or a computed tomography (CT) scan (conventional or ideally a 64-slice three-dimensional image) may be useful in evaluating changes in electrode locations or anatomy of the cochlea. Additionally, changes in a recipient's hormonal levels, which may occur during adolescence, pregnancy, menopause, or hormonal therapy (e.g., testosterone supplementation), may result in a change in electrode impedances.

Finally, a "normal" electrode impedance value does not necessarily imply that the electrode contact is in the cochlea. The clinician should remember that the electrode impedance indicates how electrical current flows across an electrode contact to surrounding tissues or fluid. A "normal" electrode impedance value may be obtained when an electrode is in contact with middle ear tissue or fluids or body tissue remote from the cochlea. Again, it is important for the programming clinician to review the cochlear implant surgeon's postoperative report and/or postoperative x-ray to determine whether all of the stimulating electrode contacts are inserted into the cochlea.

Voltage Compliance

Each cochlear implant system has a finite voltage capacity (specified by the type, number, and size of battery cells), which determines the maximum amount of current it can deliver. Ultimately, the amount of current that will be delivered to an individual electrode is determined by the efficiency of the signal delivery from the external coil to the internal device, the voltage capacity of the battery, and the electrode impedance. The aforementioned factors collectively determine the voltage compliance level of an electrode, or the maximum amount of current that can be delivered to an electrode by a given power source (e.g., battery). After stimulation reaches the voltage compliance level, additional increases in current level cannot be provided. As a result, increasing the current

level in the programming software will not result in loudness growth. If voltage compliance levels have been maximized at a value that is lower than desired, the clinician should increase the stimulus pulse width. If a recipient uses a map with electrodes that are out of voltage compliance, it is likely that speech recognition and sound quality will be compromised. Furthermore, it is probable that loudness will not be balanced across the electrode array, and the user may experience some nonauditory side effects, such as facial nerve stimulation, because the current amplitude is at a maximum.

Mixing Ratio

The mixing-ratio parameter controls the relative strength of the signal from the speech processor microphone and the direct auditory input (DAI) source. All contemporary cochlear implant sound processors have a DAI port for the direct delivery of an external input, such as a signal from a personal FM system or MP3 player, to the sound processor. In some instances, the user may desire to listen only to the signal from the DAI source (e.g., listening to music from an MP3 player). In many situations, however, a cochlear implant user will want to hear the signals from both the DAI source and sound processor microphone. For example, children using an FM system in a classroom should hear the teacher's voice from the FM transmitter, but also their own voice and the voices of other children in the room.

Typically, the mixing-ratio parameter allows the clinician to choose from a variety of ratios ranging in a graded manner from an equal emphasis on signals from the sound processor microphone and DAI (i.e., no attenuation of signal from sound processor microphone) to DAI only (i.e., complete attenuation of signal from sound processor microphone). The mixing-ratio parameter also may include the telecoil-mixing ratio, which controls the strength of the signals from the telecoil and sound processor microphone. It also ranges from equal emphasis between the telecoil and microphone signals to telecoil-only emphasis. Additional information on adjustment of the mixing ratio is provided in Chapter 7.

BASIC COCHLEAR IMPLANT SIGNAL CODING STRATEGIES

A signal coding strategy describes the algorithm used to transform the important features of the incoming acoustical signal (i.e., amplitude, frequency, and temporal cues) into an electrical code. This code attempts to represent these features in a meaningful manner to the auditory nerve. Although relatively large differences exist in the default signal coding strategies used by recent cochlear implant systems, clinical trials demonstrate comparable performance across the three systems. The following section describes contemporary cochlear implant signal coding strategies.

Continuous Interleaved Sampling (CIS)

The Continuous Interleaved Sampling (CIS) strategy is available in the cochlear implant systems for all three manufacturers, and it served as a precursor for most of the current signal coding strategies. As illustrated in Figure 2–13, the acoustic signal is sent through a bank of bandpass filters that separates the input signal into discrete frequency bands. (Note: In contemporary systems, filtering is accomplished through digital signal processing rather than physical analog filtering.) The tonotopic organization created by the filtering is preserved throughout signal processing and eventually represented to the auditory system via presentation to electrodes located in positioned

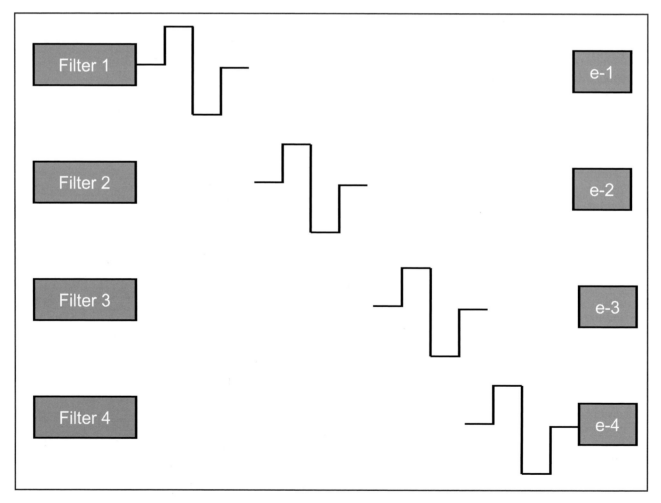

FIGURE 2–13. Illustration of the Continuous Interleaved Sampling (CIS) strategy. The acoustic signal sent through a bank of bandpass filters.

locales of the cochlea. The bandwidth of the filters varies across the three different manufacturers. The output from these filters is directed to a rectifier that converts the alternating current into a direct current signal. Following the rectifier, the signal is sent through a low-pass filter, where it is transformed into a temporal envelope. This envelope is analogous to the amplitude envelope of the acoustic input.

The CIS pulse rate must be four to five times higher than the output from the low-pass filters to prevent aliasing errors. Because early versions of CIS-type strategies used pulse rates that were less than 2,000 pps, the cut-off frequency of the low-pass filter usually is set between 200 and 400 Hz. A cut-off frequency up to 400 Hz encompasses the frequency at which the nerve can code changes in electrical pulse rate. This cut-off frequency also includes the fundamental frequency of the human voice, which is as low as 125 Hz for males and up to 400 Hz for young children.

The output of the low-pass filters is sent to a compressor that uses a logarithmic function to map the input signal into the patient's electrical dynamic range. This output from the compressor then is sent to a pulse generator, which is set to a fixed frequency. The amplitude of the pulse train from the generator is modulated on the basis of the input received from the compressor. Thus, the amplitude of the signal within each band is represented by the amplitude of the pulses within that same band. Finally, the modulated pulse trains in each channel are delivered to their respective electrode contacts.

Therefore, the intense low-frequency components of the signal are represented by high-amplitude pulses delivered to apical electrodes, while the relatively low-level, high-frequency components are represented by low-amplitude pulses delivered to the basal electrodes. All electrodes are stimulated sequentially during each stimulation cycle, and the amplitude of stimulation during each cycle corresponds to the energy present in the respective channel. Again, the frequency of the pulse trains is fixed, and stimulation occurs continuously at that stimulation frequency. Typical CIS pulse rates range from about 800 to 1,400 pps and usually are implemented with 8 to 16 channels.

Advanced Bionics offers a variation of CIS known as *Multiple Pulsatile Sampler* (MPS). MPS provides partially simultaneous stimulation. Specifically, two electrodes that are remotely spaced from one another are stimulated at the same time (i.e., electrodes 1 and 5; then 2 and 6; then 3 and 7; then 4 and 8). This approach allows for a doubling in the stimulation rate, which should theoretically improve the provision of fine temporal structural cues.

The MED-EL Corporation offers yet another variation of CIS known as CIS+ and High Definition CIS (HDCIS). CIS+ operates similarly to conventional CIS, but the frequency is expanded. Also, Hilbert transformation is used in place of wave rectification and low-pass filtering to more accurately estimate the input signal. In HDCIS, sequential stimulation between neighboring stimulation sites also is used to elicit a locus of stimulation somewhere between the two independent stimulation sites. This approach is used in an attempt to provide better spectral resolution.

HiResolution Sound Processing

HiResolution sound processing, developed by Advanced Bionics, is another variation of CIS processing. The primary differences between HiResolution and conventional CIS include (1) the provision of 16 active electrodes rather than the typical 8, (2) considerably higher maximum stimulation rates (e.g., up to 5,156 pps), (3) higher cut-off frequencies for low-pass filters (e.g., 2,800 Hz), and (4) a more sophisticated AGC system. Theoretically, the combination of the higher stimulation rates and filter cut-offs will improve the provision of fine temporal structure. An additional advantage may be the facilitation of stochastic firing in the auditory nerve that would more closely represent normal auditory nerve function.

HiResolution sound processing is available in two commercial forms, HiResS and HiResP. HiResS provides completely sequential stimulation, whereas HiResP provides partial simultaneous stimulation similar to the MPS strategy. HiResS can deliver pulse trains with rates up to 2,900 pps, while HiResP has a maximum stimulation rate of 5,156 pps. In a clinical trial, speech-recognition performance of adult recipients was significantly better with the HiRes processing when compared to conventional strategies (Koch et al., 2004). In addition, the HiRes processing was preferred by the majority of subjects.

As previously mentioned, Advanced Bionics recently released a new version of HiRes known as HiRes Fidelity 120, which incorporates current steering. Current steering attempts to increase the number of perceptual channels in the frequency domain. Through the use of current steering, HiRes Fidelity 120 creates up to 120 virtual channels. Additional channels may increase the number of frequency percepts and spectral resolution and, therefore, should improve speech recognition in noise, sound quality, and music appreciation. Results of a recent clinical trial show better speech recognition, superior sound quality ratings, and higher music appreciation when adults with Harmony processors were using the HiRes Fidelity 120 strategy compared to the HiRes strategy (Advanced Bionics Corporation, 2009). The clinician manually can convert HiRes signal coding strategies into conventional CIS or MPS signal coding strategies by disabling every other channel and selecting a wider, fixed pulse width (e.g., 75 microseconds). HiResS is converted to CIS, while HiResP is converted to MPS. Future versions of programming software likely will provide a feature that allows for automatic conversion from HiRes to CIS or MPS.

n-of-*m* Strategies

The common denominator among all of the aforementioned CIS-types strategies is that all active electrode contacts are stimulated (either in a sequential or partially simultaneous manner) for each cycle of stimulation. The *n*-of-*m* signal coding strategies utilize a different approach. For a given input sound, the acoustic energy present in each of the *m* channels is determined, and stimulation is administered to only the *n* channels with the highest amplitude inputs (Figure 2–14). The *n* is typically referred to as maxima in these types of signal coding strategies. The *n* (or maxima) typically varies from 8 to 12. Therefore, a program with 22 channels and a maxima of 10 will result in a train of biphasic pulses delivered to the 10 channels with the highest amplitude. The remaining 12 channels are not stimulated during that specific cycle.

The *n*-of-*m* strategies are designed to capture relatively low fluctuations in amplitude in the spectral domain. The reduction in the number of active electrodes during each cycle allows for (1) faster stimulation rate, (2) a reduction in channel interaction and masking, and (3) an increase in battery life. The potential limitation of *n*-of-*m* approaches is that information in some channels may not possess the necessary amplitude to be selected. As a result, the user will not have access to this acoustic information. However, research studies conducted with Cochlear Corporation users indicate that they do as well or better with an *n*-of-*m* strategy (i.e., ACE) as compared to CIS strategies (Kiefer, Hohl, Sturzebecher, Pfennigdorff, & Gstöettner, 2001; Skinner et al., 2002).

Spectral Peak (SPEAK)

SPEAK was one of the first clinically available signal coding strategies that used the *n*-of-*m* approach. The initial components are similar to that of CIS strategies. Inputs are sent through a bank of bandpass filters, in which the complex broadband sounds are divided into narrower frequency bands. The amplitude of the inputs in each channel is determined, and the *n* channels with the highest amplitudes are selected for processing. The outputs from those filters then are rectified and lowpass filtered with the cut-off frequency of 200 Hz. Finally, those outputs are used to modulate a train of biphasic pulses that are fixed in frequency (typically 250 pps) and are delivered to corresponding electrodes. In practice, the SPEAK strategy is implemented with bipolar electrode coupling in the previous generation Nucleus 22 implant and either bipolar or monopolar coupling in the Nucleus 24 and later implants. A maximum of 20 active channels are available, and the typical maxima is set at 8.

Advanced Combination Encoder (ACE)

ACE is also an *n*-of-*m* strategy that focuses on providing fine temporal structure to the user. It is similar to SPEAK, but it incorporates higher stim-

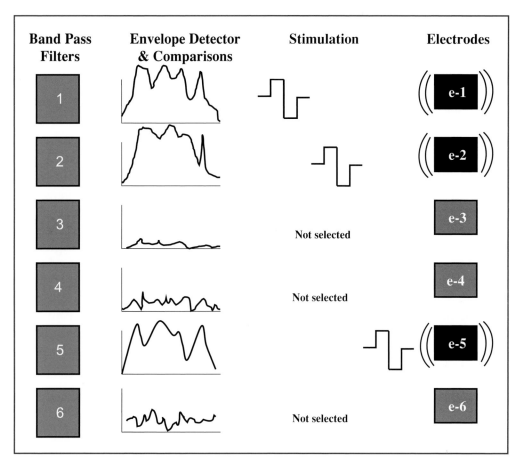

FIGURE 2–14. Block diagram of the *n*-of-*m* signal coding strategy (i.e., ACE, SPEAK). The three channels with the greatest amplitude envelopes were selected for sequential stimulation.

ulation rates. ACE is the current default signal coding strategy used with Cochlear Ltd. implants. The first version of ACE allowed for a total stimulation rate of 14,400 pps. Consequently, the per channel stimulation rate is dependent upon the number of maxima selected. If 8 maxima is selected, then a per channel rate of 1,800 pps can be achieved ($8 \times 1,800 = 14,400$). In practice, ACE uses monopolar electrode coupling. A maximum of 22 channels are available, and the typical maxima ranges from 8 to 12.

Research studies have shown that most recipients perform better with ACE than SPEAK (Kiefer et al., 2001; Skinner et al., 2002). ACE likely allows for better performance because of the provision of fine temporal structure cues via the higher stimulation rates of ACE.

Recently, Cochlear Corporation began offering a variation of ACE known as ACE(RE) or HighACE. ACE(RE) operates exactly like ACE, but the maximum total stimulation rate is 32,000 pps rather than 14,400 pps. The advantages of ACE(RE) over ACE may be negligible for many users because, as mentioned earlier, most recipients do not perform better with stimulation rates exceeding approximately 2,000 pps. In fact, in a large clinical trial, many subjects preferred and performed better with programs using rates at or below 900 pps (Arora et al., 2009; Balkany et al., 2007).

MP3000

MP3000 is yet another Cochlear Corporation variation of an *n*-of-*m* strategy. Similar to the approach used in modern MP3 recreational audio players, unimportant information in the input signal (i.e., low-level components that will be masked by adjacent higher level and more important components) is discarded. As a result, the signal is conveyed in a more efficient manner and without a significant compromise in quality or clarity.

Figure 2–15 provides a simplified illustration of the MP3000 strategy in operation. Across these 6 channels, only channels 1 and 5 will be audible for the user because the neighboring channels will be masked. As a result, stimulation is provided to only these two channels.

The primary advantage of the MP3000 strategy is an improvement in signal efficiency, which allows (proportional to the number in maxima reduction) for longer battery life, reduction in battery size, and ultimately, smaller sound processors. Preliminary research findings suggest that speech recognition with the MP3000 strategy is better than that obtained with the ACE strategy (Buchner, Nogueira, Edler, Battmer, & Lenarz,

2008). The MP3000 signal coding strategy has been used in Europe but has yet to receive FDA approval for use in the United States.

Fine Structure Processing (FSP)

MED-EL recently released a novel CIS-type signal coding strategy referred to as FSP, which has two important differences to the original CIS strategy. First, intermediate pitches are generated using bell-shaped, overlapping bandpass filters to provide better spectral resolution, which is important for the recognition of high-frequency phonemes including consonants identified on the basis of place cues (i.e., /s/, /f/, /t/). Current steering also may improve sound quality, speech recognition in noise, music appreciation, and music recognition.

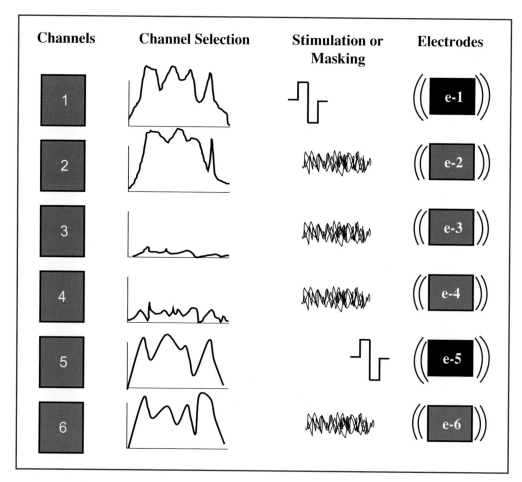

FIGURE 2–15. Illustration of MP3000 coding strategy.

The second difference from the traditional CIS strategy is that the FSP strategy modulates the timing of channel-specific sampling sequences, or pulse bursts, in the lowest frequency channels, depending on the input frequency within those channels. The conjectural advantage of this type of stimulation in the low-frequency channels is to provide better access to fine temporal structure. Additionally, it may improve speech recognition, sound quality, recognition of vocal pitch, music appreciation, and music recognition. Research on FSP is encouraging. Arnolder and colleagues (2007) report significantly improved speech and music perception with FSP relative to CIS, and most participants preferred the use of FSP over CIS.

Simultaneous Analog Stimulation (SAS)

Simultaneous Analog Stimulation (SAS) is unique when compared to the aforementioned signal coding strategies. SAS stimulates electrode contacts with continuous electrical waveforms (rather than biphasic pulses) that are analogous to the acoustical inputs to each channel. The microphone converts the acoustic input into an electrical signal, and similar to most signal coding strategies, this signal is subjected to a bank of bandpass filters. The filters separate complex electrical signals into relatively narrow frequency bands. The electrical output from each channel is subjected to compression based on a logarithmic mapping function, and then the compressed signal from each channel is sent to a dedicated electrode. Each electrode contact is stimulated at the same time (i.e., fully simultaneous stimulation) on each cycle of stimulation.

SAS has been used commercially only in Advanced Bionics cochlear implants, but it is no longer available in the current version of programming software. The typical SAS user will be an Advanced Bionics' recipient who received a cochlear implant prior to 2002. In its clinical implementation, SAS used seven to eight active electrode contacts with bipolar electrode coupling. To counter initial difficulties of avoiding voltage compliance issues, Advanced Bionics developed an internal device/electrode array that featured bipolar electrode pairs that were spaced at a greater distance than the original C1 device. The configuration of the new C1.2 device was referred to as enhanced bipolar electrode coupling.

The primary theoretical advantage of SAS is that it preserves most all of the cues present in the original input signal. The primary disadvantage is the fact that fully simultaneous stimulation likely results in a great deal of channel interaction, which may lead to distortion. Research studies examining performance differences between SAS and CIS produced mixed results (Zwolan et al., 2001). In short, this study showed that some recipients preferred and achieved at least similar performance with SAS when compared to CIS. Subjects who performed well with SAS typically had favorable preimplant histories and lower stimulation needs. Interestingly, Zwolan et al. found that recipients with the HiFocus electrode array and electrode positioner, a special component inserted along with the electrode array to facilitate proximity of the electrode contacts to the modiolus, were more likely to perform well with SAS. This finding may be attributed to the lower stimulation needs and subsequent reduction in channel interaction due to the shorter distance between the stimulating contacts and target neural elements. The electrode positioner was removed voluntarily from the market by the manufacturer in 2002 because it was associated with a higher incidence of bacterial meningitis.

KEY CONCEPTS

Following this chapter, the reader should understand the following basic terminology and concepts:

- Basic terminology is similar across cochlear implant manufacturers, but some manufacturer-specific features and signal coding strategies do exist.
- Parameters that influence coding in the intensity domain include threshold and upper stimulation levels, amplitude of current, pulse width, electrical dynamic range, IDR, sensitivity, channel gain, and volume control.

■ Parameters that influence coding in the frequency domain include the number of electrode contacts and channels, current steering, frequency allocation, and stimulation rate.

III 3 III

Basic Principles of Programming

Although some differences in cochlear implant programming exist across the three manufacturers, many more similarities can be found. It is these parallel aspects of programming that serve as the foundation for creating a good map. This chapter addresses the basic principles of cochlear implant programming that are necessary to provide a map that will optimize auditory, speech, and communication abilities as well as user satisfaction.

PRE-ACTIVATION PROCEDURES

Realistic Expectations Prior to Activation

Helping the patient and family to establish realistic expectations is one of the most important objectives prior to activation. Unfortunately, no matter how thoroughly expectations are discussed, patients and families often are discouraged with performance during the first few days or even weeks of use. This is especially true for teenagers and adults who have long periods of deafness prior to implantation. However, some adults with residual hearing and families of young children with congenital deafness also are disappointed that the implant does not provide hearing at "normal levels."

Patient dissatisfaction with initial cochlear implant use occurs for several reasons. First, the signal from a cochlear implant is much different from that of a hearing aid. Second, a period of acclimatization is required for the auditory system to adjust to the new signal. Most studies show that performance of postlingually deafened adults typically improves throughout the first one to two years of cochlear implant use (Hamzavi, Baumgartner, Pok, Franz, & Gstoettner, 2003; Oh et al., 2003). Third, most young children have little or no exposure to sound prior to implantation; consequently, a period of auditory-focused speech-language therapy normally is required before conversational, spoken-language skills emerge.

The preimplant history often determines the candidate's expectations as well as benefit and satisfaction with the implant. For example, recipients who suddenly lose hearing (e.g., ototoxic medications) have a much higher potential for immediate communicative benefit, open-set speech recognition, and successful telephone use than prelingually deafened adults. Adults who have prelingual deafness and limited open-set auditory skills are still candidates for a cochlear implant, but they will need to have realistic expectations, such as improved awareness of environmental sounds and speech-reading abilities.

Regardless of the history, counseling will help the patient understand that implant benefit will take time to manifest. Using a conservative counseling approach, audiologists should prepare adult recipients for limited word understanding and for the possibility of hearing noise for only the first few days of implant use. In reality, many adults achieve some open-set speech understanding on the first day of cochlear implant use, and as a result, they are thrilled with the early success. To enhance the counseling process, the clinician should provide written materials prior to surgery regarding realistic expectations, typical early cochlear implant outcomes, and experiences over the first year postimplant surgery (Figure 3–1). In addition, the audiologist may consider using a questionnaire, such as the measure developed by Cochlear Americas in Figure 3–2, to assess preimplant expectations and aid in counseling.

When counseling families of pediatric recipients, parents and caregivers must understand that experience and maturation is required before substantial gains are seen in a young child's communicative abilities. For example, it may take more than a year for young children without additional disabilities to develop spoken language vocabulary of even a few words. Unfortunately, approximately 40% of children with hearing loss have additional disabilities that may hinder speech and language development. Furthermore, children who are implanted at an early age (i.e., ≤1 year) may have cognitive or neurological impairments that have not been identified yet but will influence spoken language outcomes.

To prepare families of pediatric recipients and put them at ease, audiologists need to discuss all of the potential responses following activation including sound awareness, anxiety, happiness, fear, and indifference. Most children do not display a strong aversion to the experience. In fact, some are very happy with the new sound and will smile and point to their ear when they hear programming stimuli or external sounds. However, in some cases, children become upset, cry, and seek comfort from caregivers. To prevent this negative reaction, the audiologist should make every attempt to avoid overstimulation. Even with careful programming, however, a few children, especially those with minimal experience with sound, still become upset when they first hear through the implant. Finally, some children initially may be ambivalent to the sound they receive.

This response will often be concerning to the child's family because they question whether the device is working. All of these responses are possible for a young child receiving a cochlear implant, even when he or she eventually develops considerable conversational and auditory skills.

Prior to implantation, it is beneficial to provide materials that help children understand the cochlear implant process. Manufacturers offer books for young children that describe the process from surgery to activation in kid-friendly language. Also, some families create photo albums depicting their own experiences and share them with other families beginning the journey of cochlear implantation.

Reviewing Logistics of Cochlear Implantation

The audiologist should discuss the schedule of audiological, medical, and rehabilitative appointments that will be necessary for the patient before and following cochlear implantation. This discussion will prepare the family for the time and financial commitments associated with pre- and postoperative appointments. The majority of medical and audiological appointments are during the first year (i.e., diagnostic testing, programming). After the first year, medical and audiology appointments are fairly infrequent. For children, auditory-based habilitative/rehabilitative appointments are essential (e.g., one hour per week) throughout the first few years of implant use and are critically important for young children. Most adult recipients do not receive formal aural rehabilitation, but when necessary, it is usually no longer than six months following cochlear implantation.

Familiarity with Cochlear Implant Hardware

An emerging trend in cochlear implant management is to provide the patient with the external cochlear implant equipment prior to activation. This will give the adult, family, or child the opportunity to read the user manual and become acquainted with the equipment and accessories.

GENERAL INFORMATION:	ADULT: POSTLINGUAL DEAFNESS:
__General surgical considerations/risks	__If CI team recommended implant, highly likely communication ability often better than with HA
__Audiologic and rehabilitation/habilitation schedule	__Substantial variability in outcomes, outcome cannot be guaranteed
__Financial aspects: cost for surgery, audiologic & rehabilitative services, equipment, batteries, etc.	__Most score ≥ 80% sentence recognition
__Contraindications following surgery: MRI precautions, contact sports, etc.	__May not be pleased with sound quality during the first few days of use; takes some time to adjust
__Warranty policies; reliability of internal/ external equipment	__Performance often improves in first 6 mo or so
__Likelihood residual hearing eliminated by implant, potential increased risk for meningitis	__Most are able to converse over the phone __Likely more trouble than those with normal hearing in difficult environments (e.g., noise) __Self-motivation is key!
ELDERLY > 85 YRS; DURATION OF DEAFNESS:	CHILD IMPLANTED < 4 YEARS:
__Outcomes typically than obtained with hearing aids	__Outcomes vary depending on child characteristics
__Variable outcomes, may not be determined easily	__Many children develop good speech & language skills with intensive audition-based therapy
__Understanding on telephone and for TV will often improved, but may still be difficult.	__At activation, child have auditory skill of infant unless substantial residual hearing for some time
__May need longer adjustment period; reach full potential at 6 mo to ≥ 1 yr	__Post-implant, receptive lang. increase 3 mo–2 yrs; expressive lang. observed 18–30 mo
__Full-time use & frequent exposure to spoken language necessary to build auditory skill	__Post-activation, sounds have little meaning & auditory responses may be limited; time is needed for auditory skills to develop
__Post-implant aural rehabilitation is recommended for optimization of performance	__Academic Considerations
__Self-motivation & positive attitude are strong keys to success	
CHILD PRELINGUAL DEAFNESS; CI 4-7 YRS:	OLDER CHILD > 7 YRS & LIMITED SPEECH; ADULTS WITH PRELINGUAL DEAFNESS:
__If CI team recommended implant, highly likely communication ability often better than with HA	__Spoken language will always be limited compared to other populations of CI users
__Outcomes variable & dependent on many factors;	__Likely that telephone use will always be difficult
__Typically poorer outcomes than those implanted earlier; should improve sound detection	__Sound detection should improve
__Some develop speech & language skills, but likely delayed, others develop limited skills	__Initial auditory reaction may be unfavorable
__Increase in receptive lang. through 1st year; expressive lang. growth & articulation slower	__Self-motivation most important factor followed by need for intensive rehabilitation/habilitation
__Intensive audition-based therapy is critical; family must be motivated & committed	

FIGURE 3–1. Presurgery checklist for clinician to discuss with recipient about realistic expectations, typical early cochlear implant outcomes, and experiences over the first year postsurgery.

NO. 1
FAMILY/FRIEND

Cochlear

POSTLINGUISTICALLY DEAFENED
ADULT EXPECTATIONS QUESTIONNAIRE
(ANSWER TRUE or FALSE)

NAME: _____ DATE: _____

When my family member/friend receives the Nucleus Cochlear Implant.....

_____ **1.** It will be possible to carry on normal conversations when it is noisy.

_____ **2.** Music will sound normal to him/her.

_____ **3.** (S)he may need further training to make the best use of the new sounds.

_____ **4.** (S)he will understand all speech without lipreading.

_____ **5.** We may be able to have a simple conversation over the telephone.

_____ **6.** (S)he should have better control of the loudness of his/her voice.

_____ **7.** Background noise may still make communication more difficult.

_____ **8.** After listening experience, (s)he may recognize many environmental sounds.

_____ **9.** Lipreading will not be necessary at work.

_____ **10.** At first, sounds will be different than what (s)he remembers.

_____ **11.** It will be difficult for him/her to follow a conversation when several people are talking at once.

_____ **12.** (S)he will not have a hearing problem.

_____ **13.** (S)he will be assured of better job opportunities because of improved hearing.

FIGURE 3–2. Sample questions from a Cochlear America's questionnaire to assess a patient's preimplant expectations. Courtesy of Cochlear Americas, © 2003 Cochlear™ Americas.

This also will give children the chance to wear the processor without the provision of stimulation, which may put them at ease during and after the activation appointment. However, the incision site will need to be free of infection and irritation before placing the processor on the child's head. Also, some clinics recommend the use of a relatively weak magnet a day or two before the activation appointment rather than a highly magnetized transmitting coil to prevent irritation near the surgical site.

Setting the Stage

Clinicians must set the stage for success on activation day and during all programming sessions. The first consideration is the use of appropriate décor and furniture, which is especially important for young children. This action ensures optimal placement for behavioral testing and successful reinforcement with toys, distracters, snacks, and other items needed to facilitate cooperation during the session. Figure 3–3 provides examples of pediatric chairs and tables used during programming. Babies and young toddlers may be seated in a highchair during programming (Figure 3–4); however, the clinician should be aware that high-backed highchairs may interfere with the transmitting coil and knock it off the head. An effective

solution is to place a back support between the baby and the highchair back to provide support and keep the head away from the back. Highchairs with straps are helpful because they prevent the child from moving around during the potentially lengthy programming session. Figure 3–5 shows examples of seating that are conducive for older toddlers and preschool-aged children. A child-sized picnic table is also an option for children who are able to sit still and is suitable for conditioning games, coloring books, play dough, etc., used during pediatric programming sessions.

Programming sessions are often time consuming and require a great deal of concentration; therefore, it also is important that the adult recipient is comfortable throughout the session. For adults and children, the audiologist should be careful to avoid giving cues about the programming signals that are presented to the patient.

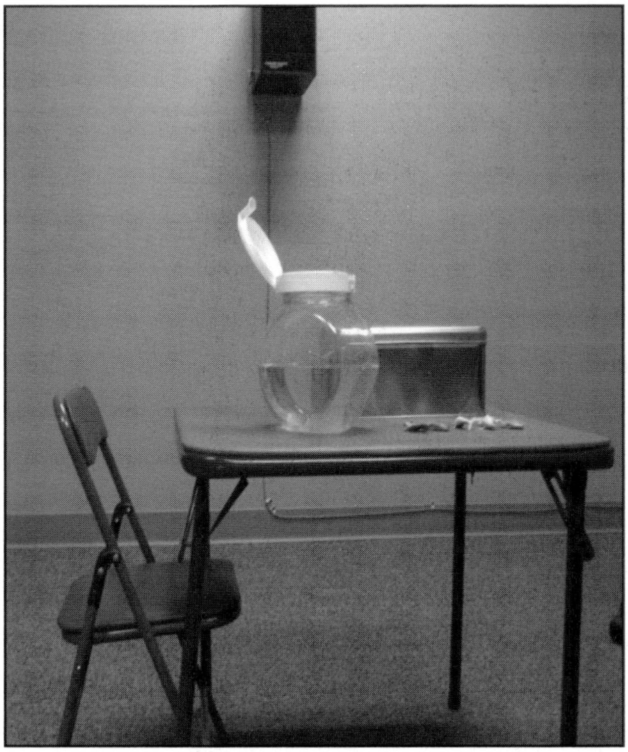

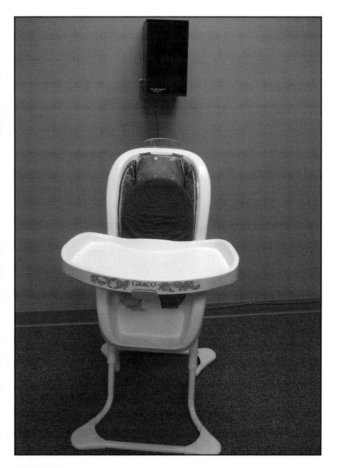

FIGURE 3–3. Examples of pediatric chair and table used during programming with fish bowl game also used for programming.

FIGURE 3–4. Highchair for use with babies and toddlers during programming.

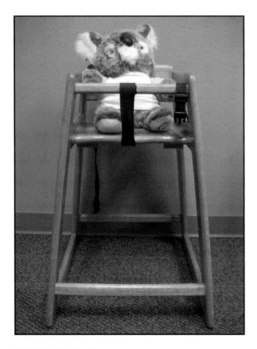 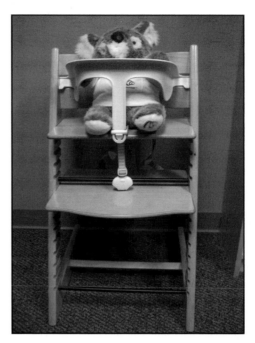

FIGURE 3–5. Examples of seating for older toddlers and early elementary children during programming.

Children, in particular, are very adept at watching the audiologist's computer monitor, hands, facial expressions, body language, etc., in an attempt to determine when they should respond to programming stimuli. Older children and adults are often seated at a 45°-angle from the audiologist and computer to avoid the detection of programming cues and to allow the clinician to observe responses. Also, the clinician should ensure that the recipient's family members are not providing cues to the user. It is not uncommon for the parent of a child to unintentionally change facial expressions or body language during the presentation of stimuli, so the programming clinician must ensure the child is not receiving augmentative cues about the programming stimuli presented during sessions.

In most cases, family members and friends should be welcome to attend programming sessions. However, if the clinician believes that the extended family and friends are preventing the recipient from focusing on the task at hand, he or she may need to request that the family members abstain from attending future appointments. Instead, a video of the session can be given to families to share with loved ones.

PROGRAMMING AFTER IMPLANTATION

Physical Evaluation

On the day of activation, the clinician needs to inspect the incision site for signs of irritation or infection and perform otoscopy on both ears. If anything remarkable (e.g., otitis media) is observed, the clinician should proceed with caution and alert the cochlear implant surgeon. Also, prior to every programming session, the clinician needs to visualize the site on which the transmitting coil rests to ensure that the magnet strength is not excessive. If a pronounced indentation and/or discoloration are present, the magnet strength should be reduced. Finally, when swelling and discomfort are alleviated around the incision site, the clinician should physically inspect the area above the internal device to ensure the device is stabilized on the desired location.

It is standard practice for the surgeon to request a postoperative x-ray to confirm that the electrode array is inserted properly. Following this imaging and prior to activation, the programming clinician needs to confer with the cochlear implant surgeon about any intracochlear electrode contacts that are not fully inserted into the cochlea. In addition, it is important to know whether any electrodes are positioned unfavorably (i.e., folded over one another) and if insertion was shallow, deep, or typical. Finally, the surgeon should inform the programming audiologist of any other pertinent details that may influence programming.

Selecting a Signal Coding Strategy

After the recipient is prepared for initial activation, the audiologist should begin by programming with the manufacturer-recommended signal coding strategy. Research has shown that some recipients perform better with one signal coding strategy over another (Pasanisi et al., 2002). Nevertheless, one type of signal coding strategy does not seem to provide optimal performance for all users. As a result, it is appropriate to allow the user to try various signal coding strategies. During the first week of implant use, the majority of recipients should be allowed to use the manufacturer-preferred signal coding strategy. However, many adults may benefit from the opportunity to experiment with alternative signal coding strategies. At least two signal coding strategies may be loaded into a patient's multiple program slots, which will permit the user to experiment with different coding strategies in real-life situations.

At the one week postactivation appointment, many adults are still acclimating to the sound from the implant and may be unable to provide detailed feedback about the different signal coding strategies. If the recipient seems overwhelmed by the new sound, it may be best to wait until the one month postactivation appointment before continuing to experiment with new strategies. Conversely, if an adult is achieving high levels of communicative success with a particular strategy and finds other strategies inferior, there is no need to continue experimenting between the preferred and new strategies.

Young children typically cannot provide reliable feedback about perceptual differences between signal coding strategies. Therefore, as a first step,

the manufacturer-recommended signal coding strategy should be used. If audiologic assessment, and more importantly, speech and language development are unfavorable, then a reasonable approach is to try an alternative signal coding strategy.

Streamlined versus Comprehensive Programming

In recent years, manufacturers have created signal coding strategies and programming platforms that expedite cochlear implant programming for two reasons. First, the number of recipients and potential candidates has increased substantially in the past decade, making it difficult for clinics to manage their expanding patient populations. Second, reimbursement for cochlear implant mapping is typically poor. Therefore, it is not financially feasible to spend a great deal of time with each recipient.

Historically, programming involved a comprehensive battery of measures to determine stimulation levels for each electrode contact in the array. In contrast, streamlined approaches involve measurements for only a few electrodes in the array. In the following paragraphs, basic programming procedures will be discussed for streamlined and comprehensive approaches.

Measuring Stimulation Levels

Recently, a great deal of attention has been given to programming parameters including stimulation rate, input dynamic range, and frequency allocation. Although these parameters clearly can impact performance, the most important aspect of programming is the optimization of stimulus levels. The following section discusses the various procedures used to determine appropriate stimulation levels for adults and children.

Setting Threshold Levels for Adults

Setting the threshold of electrical stimulation (i.e., T level) for an adult recipient is important because it determines the amount of stimulation necessary to restore audibility and normalize loudness for low-level sounds. In most cases, procedures for determining T levels are similar to those used to obtain routine audiometric thresholds. However, as previously mentioned, research has suggested that many adults with contemporary Advanced Bionics and MED-EL cochlear implants experience good outcomes and have sufficient audibility for low-level sounds when T levels are set to zero or estimated on the basis of the upper stimulation level (Spahr & Dorman, 2005).

Testing often begins on a low-frequency channel because listeners with hearing loss are more likely to recognize a stimulus that was familiar prior to surgery (i.e., most individuals had some low-frequency hearing prior to surgery). The low-frequency stimuli should be presented at a level that is clearly audible, but not uncomfortable, to give recipients a reference for the stimulus they are trying to detect. After audibility is established, traditional threshold testing begins using an adaptive-bracketing procedure, such as the modified Hughson-Westlake (Carhart & Jerger, 1959). Recipients may respond to lower stimulation levels for descending presentations as compared to ascending presentations. Therefore, to ensure audibility of soft acoustic inputs, T levels should be based on responses acquired in the ascending direction.

The step size for ascending and descending presentations varies. Assessment of precise T levels at the initial activation can be difficult because recipients are not accustomed to the signal from the implant, and therefore, may respond at only supratheshold levels. Because the user's T-level responses are likely to change over the first few weeks of cochlear implant use, the clinician should use larger step sizes for the first few appointments. After a week or more of implant use, the "internal noise" or tinnitus in the auditory system typically diminishes, and the adult recipient is much more adept at responding to signals at true T level. As a result, step size typically is decreased to provide a more precise measure of the electrical threshold.

Using the computer/processor interface, the audiologist presents a train of biphasic pulses to the external sound processor at a stimulation rate equal to what is used in the recipient's program. The audiologist asks the recipient to indicate whether he or she detects the stimulus by saying "yes" or raising a hand. The exact definition of T level varies across manufacturers, but as a general rule, T level is set to 50% threshold level (or just below) for CIS-type strategies and to the minimum amount of stimulation necessary for 100% detection for *n*-of-*m* strategies. As previously mentioned, T levels should be determined according to two responses obtained in an ascending presentation mode.

After establishing the T level on a given channel, the clinician should proceed to another electrode located toward a more basal portion of the array (i.e., mid- and then high-frequency channels). If the recipient fatigues during the measurement of T levels, the clinician could estimate T levels across the electrode array on the basis of measurements made at different points throughout the array (i.e., interpolation).

At follow-up programming appointments, the clinician should be fairly confident with the recipient's T levels based on previous programming sessions. Therefore, the clinician may begin testing below the expected threshold of audibility to improve efficiency and to avoid the use of suprathreshold presentation levels. To prevent any confusion, however, an audible reference stimulus may be given prior to testing. T levels should be measured several times during the first year of cochlear implant use. Research has shown that T levels of adults increase slightly over the first two months of use and typically are stable from that point forward (Hughes et al., 2001). After an adult recipient has a stable cochlear implant program and is performing well, evaluation and programming should occur one to two times per year. A suggested programming and evaluation schedule for adult implant recipients is provided in Chapter 5.

Negative consequences may arise when T levels are not programmed appropriately. When set too low, the recipient will not have adequate audibility of low-level or soft sounds. When set too high (i.e., above the real threshold), the subject may hear too much ambient noise, and the electrical dynamic range will be reduced unnecessarily. Reduction of an already limited electrical dynamic range will make it even harder for the audiologist to accommodate the wide range of typical acoustic inputs and desired loudness experiences. Also, when T levels are set too high in CIS-type strategies, the user may report a continuous noise that sounds like "bacon frying," "buzzing," "hissing," or "static."

In addition to traditional threshold measurement techniques (i.e., modified Hughson-Westlake), three other approaches can be taken for determining T levels: (1) the count-the-beep method, (2) psychophysical loudness scaling, and (3) threshold estimation. The count-the-beep method uses a gated stimulus and often is selected for recipients who have difficulty distinguishing between their tinnitus and a continuous programming stimulus. When using this approach, the patient is asked to count the number of programming stimuli that were arbitrarily selected and presented by the clinician. The T level corresponds to the stimulus level that results in 100% accuracy. Skinner, Holden, Holden, and Demorest (1995) showed that use of the count-the-beep method for setting T levels results in better access to low-level sounds when compared to programs created via the audiometric-style approach.

The second alternative procedure for establishing T levels, psychophysical loudness scaling, determines the stimulation level corresponding to a soft-loudness percept. Using a chart for assessing loudness growth, the clinician gradually increases the presentation level starting at a point that is inaudible and eventually stops when the stimulus level is perceived as "loud." T level is set to the stimulus level that corresponds to a psychophysical rating of "soft." When comparing traditional and loudness scaling methods, Skinner and colleagues (1995) concluded that programs established using loudness scaling resulted in better access to soft sounds for recipients of the Nucleus 22 cochlear implant and Spectra body-worn sound processor. Because input-processing characteristics and mapping functions have improved relative to the technology that was available in the Spectra processor, audibility of low-level inputs is often sufficient with T levels set using an audiometric-style approach. However, the psychophysical loudness scaling approach may be beneficial for users with abnormally slow loudness growth over the lower portion of their electrical dynamic range (e.g., all stimuli from 125–155 clinical units are perceived as soft) and fast for the upper portion (e.g., 155–165 clinical units equals the percept ranging from soft to loud, but comfortable). Limited loudness growth over a substantial portion of the lower electrical dynamic range sometimes is described as a "T-tail," which refers to the limited change in loudness percept across a wide range of stimulation levels. When a T-tail occurs, it often is helpful to increase T levels to the point at which loudness begins to grow with increases in stimulus level. Detection of T-tails and the point at which loudness begins to grow above threshold can be identified using only the psychophysical scaling method.

The final alternative method for determining T levels is through the use of manufacturer-developed estimation strategies. T levels are estimated on the basis of the user's upper stimulation levels, typical electrical dynamic ranges with those upper stimulation levels, and logarithmic mapping functions that aim to place the majority of acoustic inputs into the upper portion of the electrical dynamic range. Research has shown that most recipients achieve adequate audibility for low-level sounds when T levels are estimated from upper stimulation levels (Spahr & Dorman, 2005). However, for patients who have atypically narrow electrical dynamic ranges, T levels should be measured manually to ensure audibility for low-level sounds.

Setting Threshold Levels for Children

Setting electrical-threshold levels in children may be a challenge; however, T levels can be accurately established for most children by using traditional, age-appropriate methods to determine audiometric thresholds. These techniques include behavioral observation audiometry (BOA), visual reinforcement audiometry (VRA), conditioned play audiometry (CPA), and the standard audiometric approach used for adults. The success of a particular technique is dependent on the chronological and developmental age, mood and behavior, and listening experience of the child as well as the conditioning, reinforcement strategies, and skill level of the programming assistant.

Regardless of the technique, an animated and enthusiastic programming test assistant is essential for obtaining valid results. It is almost impossible for a single person to program a cochlear implant sound processor, manage a child's behavior, and facilitate cooperation during a lengthy programming session. Many clinics designate an audiologist as the programmer and a second audiologist or a speech-language therapist as the test assistant. Children will be particularly comfortable with the speech-language pathologist or Listening and Spoken Language Specialist (LSLS) whom they see on a weekly basis. Also, the LSLS can practice the CPA response (i.e., drop the toy in the bucket when stimulus heard) in weekly therapy sessions to encourage cooperation during audiology appointments. Other clinics may use trained support personnel as the programming assistant. All of these options are viable as long as the assistant is familiar with the objective of the task and adept at managing the behavior of the child. The job of the test assistant is to facilitate a conditioned response from the child, keep the child engaged, ensure the transmitting coil remains on the head, manage the child's behavior, assist in objective measures (i.e., electrically evoked stapedial reflex threshold), and help in observing the child's responses.

In pediatric audiology, BOA has long been considered an unreliable method of determining the threshold of audibility of a young child. Recently, however, Jane Madell (2008) described a unique variation of BOA for infants (0 to 6 months) that provides a more reliable and valid measure of behavioral threshold. Briefly, the Madell approach involves the observation of a change in the child's sucking pattern when listening to test stimuli. To aid in the success of the measure, Madell recommends that the child is hungry upon arrival to an appointment. A pacifier then is inserted into the child's mouth, and test stimuli are presented. Detection of a stimulus is noted when a time-locked sucking pattern changes (i.e., cessation or initiation of sucking). The authors have used this approach successfully to measure T levels and soundfield cochlear implant detection thresholds in young children (9 to 15 months).

Traditional VRA testing techniques are optimal for determining T levels in children with a developmental age ranging from 10 to 20 months. As a result, it is imperative that pediatric cochlear implant clinics have VRA equipment in sound-field test booths and programming rooms.

Traditional CPA testing techniques are suitable for measuring T levels in children with developmental ages ranging from 18 months to 8 years. Although 18 months is traditionally younger than expected for this task, the authors have worked with children who develop a conditioned play response prior to 18 months of age. Some older children (≥6 years) will prefer a conventional audiometric approach, while others will not be able to maintain attention over long periods of time. Therefore, clinicians should be flexible and use the approach that yields the most reliable and valid threshold responses for a particular child.

One factor that influences the success of CPA is a child's interest in the variety of activities, toys, and games used during testing. Because children with cochlear implants must attend multiple programming sessions and audiometric evaluations per year, it is critical to provide a variety of exciting and entertaining CPA tasks. Figure 3–6 provides several examples of CPA games proven successful for establishing T levels. For young children or those who are inattentive and hyperactive, it may be necessary to use multiple CPA toys during the session.

The same ascending/descending approach used to measure thresholds in adults also is applicable to young children. However, for young children with shorter attention spans, larger step sizes may be used to obtain T levels. Also, similar to adult procedures, measurement of T levels should begin with a low-frequency (i.e., apical) electrode contact. When a valid threshold is obtained for a low-frequency contact, the clinician should promptly move on to an electrode contact in the middle of the array, followed by a basal electrode contact. If the child's attention is maintained, T levels should be obtained on as many electrodes as possible. Interpolation is used to estimate T levels on unmeasured channels.

At initial activation, the child's T levels are likely above the true threshold. Thus, it may be necessary to provide a slight decrease in the T levels for the child's map. T levels in children appear to increase rather significantly through the first few months of implant use and stabilize by 3 months to 1-year post implantation (Henkin et al., 2006;

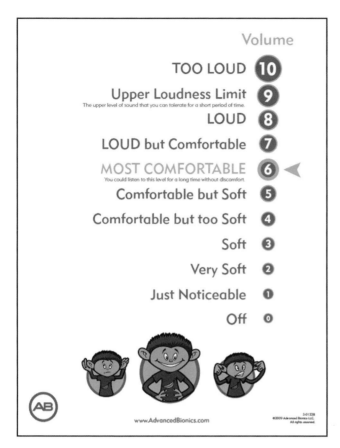

Volume

TOO LOUD (10)

Upper Loudness Limit (9)
The upper level of sound that you can tolerate for a short period of time.

LOUD (8)

LOUD but Comfortable (7)

MOST COMFORTABLE (6) ◄
You could listen to this level for a long time without discomfort.

Comfortable but Soft (5)

Comfortable but too Soft (4)

Soft (3)

Very Soft (2)

Just Noticeable (1)

Off (0)

FIGURE 3–6. Example of an Advanced Bionics loudness scale for determining electrical threshold with adults. Courtesy of Advanced Bionics (http://www.Advanced Bionics.com).

Henkin, Kaplan-Neeman, Muchnik, Kronenberg, & Hildesheimer, 2003; Hughes et al., 2001). After the first 6 months of implant use, the authors recommend that young children return for evaluation and programming on a quarterly basis to ensure that T levels are appropriate.

By no later than 1 month postactivation, the clinician should measure the child's minimal response levels in the soundfield to frequency-specific stimuli. Responses should be no greater than 30 dB HL in the low frequencies and should not exceed 25 dB HL in the mid to high frequencies. If the child's responses do not meet these criteria, the clinician should seek to optimize T-level stimulation through manual adjustments (see Chapters 4 and 5).

Manufacturer-developed, threshold-estimation procedures may be used with children only when their upper stimulation levels are optimized. In general, the authors recommend manual measurement of threshold with children to ensure adequate stimulation for low-level inputs. Psychophysical loudness scaling procedures for setting T levels also are not recommended for children because the task often is too difficult for them to perform. However, given the sensitivity of loudness scaling for detecting T-tails and the point at which loudness begins to grow above threshold, clinicians need to be sensitive and aware of two red flags. First, if a child has an unusually large electrical dynamic range, and the clinician is certain upper stimulation levels are set appropriately, it is probable that loudness growth is very shallow in the lower part of the electrical dynamic range. As a result, it may be helpful to provide a global increase in T levels across the electrode array. A global change in stimulation refers to increasing or decreasing stimulation across all channels by the same amount. The clinician also should be attentive for signs of insufficient access to low-level sounds. If the child's caregivers or LSLS reports that the child does not consistently respond to soft sounds, it may be necessary to increase T levels. Finally, if soundfield detection thresholds are elevated, T levels should be increased to provide better access to low-level sounds. Prior to adjustment of T levels, the clinician should verify that elevated soundfield thresholds are not related to a faulty microphone. Malfunctioning microphones typically cause greater elevation for high-frequency sounds.

One streamlined approach to measuring T levels is to provide gradual and global increases to T levels across the electrode array until the child responds to speech and environmental sounds. However, this approach should be used as a last resort because T levels are likely to vary across the electrode array. Therefore, based on crude responses to environmental stimuli, global changes to T levels likely will result in insufficient settings for some channels.

Additional Measure to Ensure Adequate T Levels and Confirm Audibility

For children and adults, many clinicians ensure adequate audibility for sounds across the speech frequency range by confirming that the recipient can detect all six Ling sounds (/ah/, /oo/, /ee/, /s/, /sh/, and /m/; Ling, 1976, 1989). These six phonemes encompass the typical range of speech frequencies, so audibility for the Ling sounds should ensure audibility for most speech sounds. During the first few days of implant use, all six Ling sounds should be audible when spoken at an average conversational level, 6 feet away from the user. By 1 month of implant use, all six Ling sounds should be audible when spoken at a distance of at least 15 feet from the user. Furthermore, a goal of accurate discrimination of all six Ling sounds should be rapidly pursued, and on a daily basis, the parents of young children should ensure that the child can hear all six Ling sounds.

Setting Upper Stimulation Levels for Adults

The provision of optimal upper stimulation levels (i.e., M, MCL, or C levels depending on manufacturer) is one of the most challenging aspects of the programming process. Even with adults, it can be difficult to determine exactly where upper stimulation levels should be set across the electrode array in order to provide optimal sound quality and speech recognition. Underestimating the upper stimulation levels may sacrifice speech recognition, hamper sound quality, and limit self-monitoring abilities of the recipient's voice (i.e., intensity, vocal quality). Overestimating stimulation levels may cause discomfort, hinder speech recognition, influence sound quality, and foster an aversive reaction to the implant.

Similar to T levels, the maximum level of stimulation that a recipient will tolerate is likely to change over the first few months of cochlear implant use. Many users are able to reach a desired level of stimulation for optimal performance after several weeks of cochlear implant use. However, some recipients will require gradual changes to reach an optimal upper stimulation level. In only rare exceptions are adults comfortable with appropriate upper stimulation levels during the first week of implant use. Most importantly, recipients differ in what they initially will tolerate. The clinician must balance the impor-

tance of an optimal cochlear implant program with the prevention of overstimulation in the early stages of implant use.

One popular method to measure upper stimulation levels is via psychophysical loudness scaling. To begin this procedure, the programming stimulus is presented to an electrode contact or to a band of channels, and the recipient is asked to indicate the loudness percept of the stimulus by pointing to a loudness scaling chart (Figure 3–7). The clinician gradually increases the level of the programming stimulus until the recipient reports that it is comfortably loud. This process is repeated for many, if not all, of the electrode contacts in the array. If upper stimulation levels are not measured for each individual electrode contact, interpolation is used to set the levels of the unmeasured electrode contacts.

Another approach to setting upper stimulation levels is to provide a global increase in upper stimulation levels while the user listens to live speech. The upper stimulation levels will be set where speech and environmental sounds are most comfortable. Some clinicians also will choose to then tilt or provide tapered decreases or increases in the low- or high-frequency portion of the array to address patient complaints or comments regarding sound quality. For instance, if the recipient reports that sounds have too much bass or are too sharp, the clinician can taper off the upper stimulation levels in the low or high frequencies, respectively. On the other hand, if a recipient cannot hear his or her voice very well or if speech lacks sufficient clarity, the clinician may increase upper stimulation levels in the low or high frequencies, respectively.

A third and more objective approach to setting upper stimulation levels is the use of electrically evoked stapedial reflex thresholds (ESRT). Many clinicians use ESRT as a standard component of their programming test battery because it is a straightforward and simple measure to administer. First, the clinician places an acoustic immittance probe into the external ear canal contralateral to the cochlear implant. Second, he or she continuously records the acoustic admittance, set to a 226 Hz probe tone, while presenting the programming stimulus for obtaining upper stimulation level to

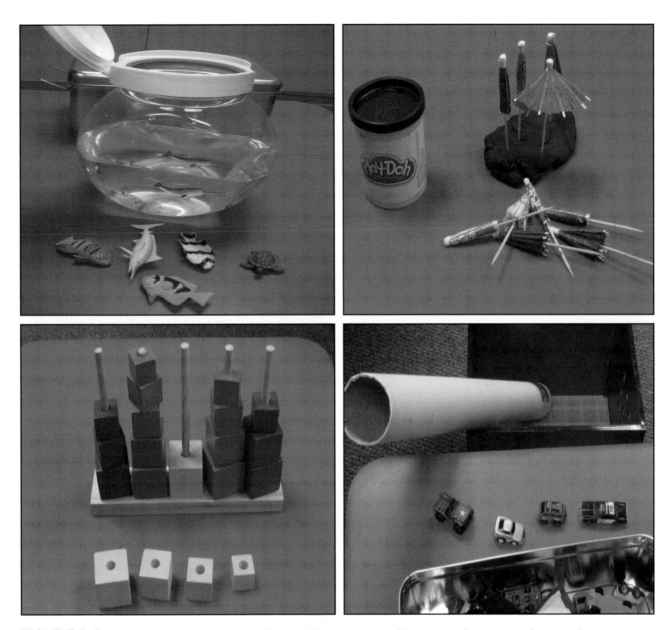

FIGURE 3–7. Examples of games used for conditioned play audiometry and programming sessions.

the cochlear implant in an ascending manner. When the level of the stimulus from the implant is sufficiently intense to elicit the stapedial reflex, the clinician observes a decrease in admittance, which is time-locked with stimulus presentations (Figure 3–8). This decrease in admittance can be observed in the ear contralateral to the cochlear implant because the stapedial reflex is a bilateral response. It actually is recommended that the immittance probe be placed in the contralateral

ear as the response is more likely to be measured in an ear that is unaltered by surgery.

The ESRT is measured on as many channels as possible, and remaining channels are set via interpolation. Initially, upper stimulation levels are set according to the ESRT and then are decreased globally below the patient's uncomfortable loudness level. Next, the upper stimulation levels gradually are increased globally while the recipient listens to speech and environmental sounds

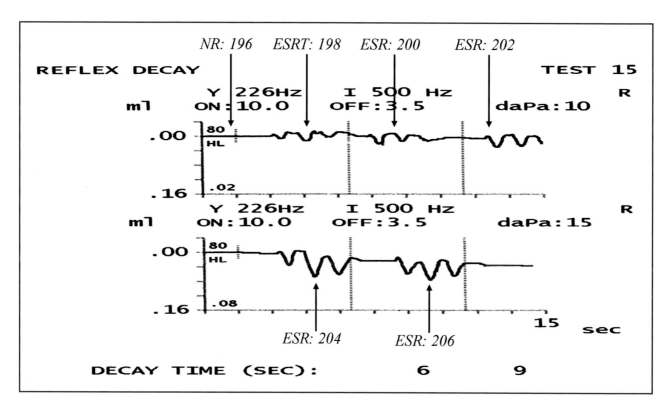

FIGURE 3–8. Visual display of the ESRT obtained with a cochlear implant recipient.

in live speech mode to a level that corresponds to a comfortably loud rating. However, the upper stimulation levels are not set higher than the ESRT. Doing so likely would result in continuous elicitation of the stapedial reflex threshold to moderately intense sounds, such as average conversational speech. This is not typical for persons with normal hearing and should not be a reality for cochlear implant users. Adults who used high-power hearing aids for many years frequently will desire upper stimulation levels that are excessively high, but setting the upper stimulation levels at erroneously high levels may hamper performance. In these cases, the ESRT can serve as a limit for upper stimulation levels.

Published reports suggest ESRT is measurable in approximately 65 to 85% of implant users (Battmer, Laszig, & Lehnhardt, 1990; Brickley et al., 2005; Gordon, Papsin, & Harrison, 2004); however, it is not present for all recipients. Subtle middle-ear anomalies are likely responsible for the inability to measure the response in approxi-

mately 30% of recipients. If the response is not present in the contralateral ear, the measurement may be attempted in the ipsilateral ear. Unfortunately, an ipsilateral response may not be present because the cochlear implant surgery may result in subtle fixation of the middle-ear system.

Several research studies show that the ESRT is an excellent predictor of upper stimulation levels (Brickley et al., 2005; Jerger, Oliver, and Chmiel, 1988). In fact, correlation coefficients between ESRT and upper stimulation levels are strong and range from .79 to .85 (Brickley et al.; Hodges et al., 1997; Lorens, Walkowiak, Piotrowska, Skarzynski, & Anderson, 2004). Recipients also will perceive equal loudness when upper stimulation levels are based on ESRT assessments (Hodges et al.). Balancing of loudness across the electrode array should result in optimal sound quality and speech recognition. In fact, programs that are based on ESRT often result in higher sound-quality ratings and similar or better speech-recognition performance when compared to programs based on conventional psychophysical loudness assessments (Hodges et al.; Spivak, Chute, Popp, & Parisier, 1994; Wolfe & Kasulis, 2008).

Setting Upper Stimulation Levels for Children

The ESRT is the highly recommended procedure for setting upper stimulation levels in children, and clinicians always should attempt to complete this measure with pediatric recipients. ESRT is crucial in determining optimal upper stimulation levels because psychophysical loudness measures typically are not feasible for children until they are at least 4 years old. Furthermore, precise measures of loudness are not achievable until approximately 8 years of age.

Similar to adults, research supports the use of ESRT for predicting upper stimulation levels for children. Typically, the ESRT is within an average of nine clinical units of upper stimulation levels (Spivak & Chute, 1994) and are often lower than upper stimulation-level settings based on behavioral measures (Bresnihan, Norman, Scott, & Viani, 2001). In other words, when using behavioral measures, clinicians often have a tendency to overestimate comfort levels of children. Because of the improved comfort of ESRT-based programs, children often will use their cochlear implants for longer periods of time and experience fewer episodes of discomfort to speech and environmental sounds (Bresnihan et al., 2001). Some clinicians will be compelled to slowly increase upper stimulation levels for children over time (Zwolan, O'Sullivan, Fink, Niparko, & CDACI Investigative Team, 2008), but the clinician will need to use extreme caution to avoid the provision of excessively high upper stimulation levels. A more objective approach for setting upper stimulation levels is to use ESRT as a guide, which will avoid overstimulating a child and should provide better performance with the implant.

In the event that the ESRT cannot be recorded, the clinician must rely on behavioral measures to determine upper stimulation levels. For children who are preschool-aged and younger, this almost invariably means using behavioral observation of reactions following stimulation. To begin this procedure, stimulation to a channel or band of channels is increased gradually as the behavior of the child is monitored by the programming audiologist, programming assistant, and caregivers. Typically, it is ideal to have the child engaged in a mildly entertaining task while this occurs (e.g., looking at toys, watching television, etc.). When the child begins to exhibit signs that the stimulus is too loud, the clinician should immediately stop the programming stimulus. These signs are often subtle and include holding his or her breath; exhibiting facial expressions of mild concern; looking to a caregiver for reassurance; tensing or stiffening of the body or shoulders; playing more actively or aggressively; wringing hands, clothes, or toys; and producing blinks in response to the stimulus. It is critically important to observe these signs as they are an indication of mild discomfort. Continuing to increase the stimulation level eventually will lead to overstimulation, an adverse reaction, and a negative association with the cochlear implant. If this occurs, it may be difficult to convince the child to wear the sound processor during the early stages.

For older children (≥4 years), upper stimulation level may be set via simplified psychophysical-loudness approaches as described by Serpanos and Gravel (2002). Figure 3–9 shows an example of a basic loudness scaling card, which based on the authors' experience, is used successfully with preschool and elementary-aged children. Children who are 8 to 9 years old and good readers often can participate in the traditional psychophysical loudness scaling procedures.

To avoid overstimulation, the clinician should never activate the implant to live speech at the initial upper stimulation levels because of channel summation. Therefore, after upper stimulation levels are set to programming stimuli, they are decreased globally well below the child's uncomfortable loudness level (i.e., slightly above or even below the minimum response level). The implant then may be activated in live speech mode, and the upper stimulation levels may be increased globally while the child is listening to speech and environmental sounds. Once again, the clinicians and the caregivers should look for signs of subtle aversive responses. When these signs are observed,

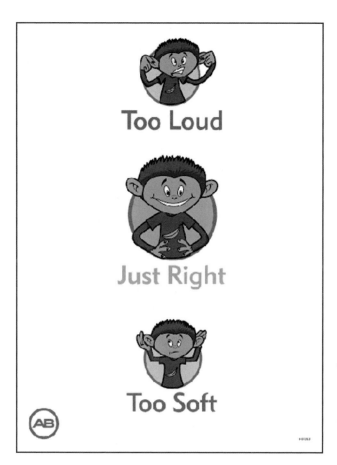

FIGURE 3–9. Advanced Bionics loudness scaling card for young children. Courtesy of Advanced Bionics (http://www.AdvancedBionics.com).

the upper stimulation levels should be decreased globally and gradually to a level that is comfortable for the child.

While adjusting upper stimulation levels in live speech mode, it may be helpful for children to play with noise makers (e.g., drum sticks, xylophones, tambourines). Typically, when upper stimulation levels are set too low, children will play the noise makers enthusiastically and create sounds that are excessively loud. However, when the upper stimulation levels approach an uncomfortable level, children will stop playing vigorously with the noise makers or will start blinking to any sharp or loud sounds the noise makers produce. The upper stimulation level should be set below the level that elicits these behavioral changes and at a level that is obviously tolerable by the child.

Additional Measures to Set Stimulation Levels

Two additional measures to enhance user performance and sound quality include loudness balancing and electrode sweeping. Loudness balancing involves the confirmation that the loudness percept is equivalent across the electrode array when programming stimuli are presented at a specified level within the electrical dynamic range. This measure is recommended for older children (≥7 years) and adults when ESRT cannot be obtained. To implement this simple procedure, the standard programming stimulus is presented at the upper stimulation level to the most apical channel (e.g., channel 22) and to the neighboring channel (e.g., channel 21). If the subject perceives equal loudness in the two channels, the clinician repeats the task for channels 21 and 20. However, if the subject reports that one of the channels is louder, the clinician will slightly adjust the level of the second channel in the pair (i.e., Channel 21) and will repeat the task until equal loudness is achieved between the two channels. Figure 3–10 shows an example of a loudness-balancing card that may be used during the procedure. The adjustment to the stimulation level always should be to the second electrode in the pair because the first electrode is balanced to the preceding electrodes in the array. Some clinicians may attempt to assess loudness balance across three to four channels at a time, but the recipient typically will find the task more manageable when it is restricted to two channels at a time. On occasion, clinicians will adjust T levels to achieve loudness balance at the lower end of the electrical dynamic range (e.g., 25 or 50%). However, in the authors' experience, loudness balancing should be confined to upper stimulation levels because the T levels already are set appropriately using reliable and valid measures or estimation; therefore, they should not be adjusted.

Balancing loudness at the upper stimulation levels is important for several reasons. First, when the upper stimulation levels in one channel are perceived as much louder than the other channels, the overall loudness percept will be influenced significantly. As a result, when listening in live speech mode, the recipient will seek to decrease

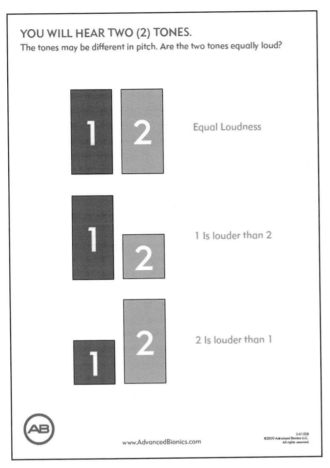

FIGURE 3–10. Advanced Bionics chart that may be used during loudness-balancing procedure. Courtesy of Advanced Bionics (http://www.AdvancedBionics.com).

the upper stimulation levels globally to account for the one channel that is excessively loud. Second, equal loudness at upper stimulation levels across the array yields optimal speech recognition. If certain channels have inadequate loudness, the speech cues within those channels will not be salient, and the interphoneme loudness relationship may be skewed. Finally, balancing loudness across the array provides optimal sound quality for the recipient. Given these reasons, the clinician should strive to ensure loudness balancing for all recipients whether it is determined with the behavioral procedure or through ESRT.

Some recipients find the loudness-balancing task very difficult because it requires the detection of subtle variations in loudness and pitch that occur when stimuli are presented across channels. This is especially true for assessments at the basal (i.e., high frequency) end of the array and when working with younger children who have not fully developed the concepts of loudness and pitch. However, it is an essential component of programming when ESRT cannot be measured.

The second procedure that may be used to improve the determination of upper stimulation levels is electrode sweeping. When implementing this procedure, the programming stimulus is presented sequentially or swept across all electrode contacts in the array beginning at the apical end and ending at the base. Three objectives are associated with electrode sweeping: (1) measuring sound quality, (2) determining appropriate pitch transitions, and (3) confirming equal loudness across channels. Sweeping to evaluate sound-quality issues is not performed at every mapping session, but it is a good practice for newly implanted recipients or for those experiencing difficulties that cannot be resolved with conventional mapping techniques or troubleshooting of the external equipment.

A determination of sound quality is performed by asking the recipient to listen to a stimulus and report whether any of the stimuli have poor sound quality (i.e., noise). Normally, the stimulus should possess a tonal percept, but if the user reports hearing noise, experiences pain or other unwanted sensations, has facial nerve stimulation, or simply reports poor sound quality, the clinician may consider disabling or adjusting the stimulation on the contact.

Secondly, the clinician may use electrode sweeping to ensure that the recipient perceives an orderly and expected transition in pitch as stimulation is swept from the apical (i.e., low pitch) to the basal (i.e., high pitch) portion of the array. If the expected tonotopic organization is not observed, the clinician may either disable or reallocate the anomalous electrodes to different channels. Management of this rare problem is discussed in Chapters 4 and 6.

Finally, sweeping may be used to confirm equal loudness across the entire array rather than the traditional two to three electrodes at a time (i.e., loudness balancing). When using this procedure, the clinician instructs the recipient to listen to all of the stimuli and raise a hand if any sounds are substantially softer or louder than the rest. This task may be performed at upper stimulation levels or at lower portions of the electrical dynamic range.

Adjustments to Special Parameters

Stimulation Rate

As mentioned in Chapter 2, a great deal of interest exists in how stimulation rate affects performance. Most recipients achieve maximum performance with stimulation rates that exceed a few hundred pulses per second (pps), but considerable individual variation exists. Contemporary cochlear implants allow the clinician to select between stimulation rates varying from a few hundred to several thousand pps.

A paucity of well-controlled, large studies indicate substantial benefit for stimulation rates exceeding approximately 3,000 pps for the majority of subjects, and some recipients actually show detrimental effects to high stimulation rates. Because sound clinical decisions should be based on evidence-based research, an initial stimulation rate less than or equal to 3,000 pps is recommended. The exact initial stimulation rate is specific to each cochlear implant system (i.e., make and model) and is provided in Chapter 4.

Regardless of the initial stimulation rate, recipients should be given the opportunity to try multiple stimulation rates, especially if they are not satisfied with the initial setting. In most cases, the recipient's unsophisticated auditory-skill level with the cochlear implant may not facilitate valid comparisons between stimulation rates. However, at some point between the 1-week and 1-month post-activation programming session, the user should be experienced enough to indicate which stimulation rate is preferable. During this comparison process, the clinician may allow the user to listen to programs with a range of stimulation rates (i.e., 500, 1,500, 3,000 pps). In many instances, a patient is able to make an unequivocal decision about the preferred stimulation rate. If a recipient is wavering between two different rates, the clinician can create a program for each rate, which will allow the user to experiment during daily situa-

tions. The recipient then can select the preferred rate at a follow-up appointment in 1 month.

It is often impossible for young children to provide reliable feedback about various stimulation rates. For pediatric programming, the clinician ought to begin with the stimulation rate that is best supported by clinical research or the manufacturer's recommendation. Device-specific recommendations are provided in Chapter 4. Clinicians should experiment with stimulation rate in young children only when expected progress is not achieved.

Pulse Width

When the desired current level is hindered by voltage constraints of the cochlear implant system, the pulse width may be increased (i.e., widened). However, an inverse relationship exists between pulse width and stimulation rate. Higher stimulation rates require a narrower pulse width. Therefore, if a patient requires high levels of stimulation, the pulse width may have to be increased. As a result, the stimulation rate will have to be decreased. The exact manner in which stimulation rate and pulse width are managed varies slightly from one cochlear implant system to another and are discussed in detail in Chapter 4.

Channel Gain

Channel gain affects the intensity of the signal before it is processed by the external sound processor. After the clinician ensures that stimulation levels are optimized for recipients using CIS-type strategies, adjustments to channel gain may address subtle sound quality complaints or speech recognition difficulties. For instance, if upper stimulation levels are set as high as a patient can tolerate, but he or she still complains of muffled speech, channel gains may be increased in the high frequencies. Additionally, if a recipient reports that his or her own voice is too soft and low-frequency upper-stimulation levels cannot be increased without exceeding the voltage limits of the device, the clinician may increase low-frequency channel gains to enhance the loudness. Furthermore, to improve speech recognition and comfort in noise, the clinician may create a program that includes decreased gains in the low-frequency channels. In reality, when stimulation levels are set appropriately, there is usually no need to adjust channel gains. Finally, as will be discussed further in Chapter 5, gains should be adjusted as a last resort in *n*-of *m*-type strategies.

Frequency Allocation

Frequency allocation is particularly relevant when one or more electrodes must be disabled. In the Advanced Bionics system, it is determined automatically and is not a clinician-adjustable parameter. However, in the Cochlear Corporation and MED-EL devices, the clinician can control how frequencies are allocated to electrodes, but significant differences exist in the way this parameter is adjusted between the two systems (see Chapter 4).

When electrodes are disabled, the bandwidth of each channel becomes wider, but the overall range of input frequencies remains the same. Wider channel bandwidths may result in processing of two different frequencies within the same channel, which will make them sound similar. As a result, narrower channel bandwidths are preferable. According to research, restricting the upper end of the input frequency range from about 10,000 Hz to approximately 8,000 Hz resulted in narrower channel bandwidths across the speech frequencies and improved speech recognition (Skinner, Holden, & Holden, 1995, 1997). Because disabling electrodes may influence frequency allocation and performance, it should be done only when absolutely necessary. Disabling may be necessary when an electrode has abnormal electrode impedance values, elicits undesired nonauditory side effects (e.g., facial nerve stimulation, pain), or possesses a poor auditory response relative to other electrodes.

The total range of frequencies allocated for adults should extend out to at least 6,000 Hz to allow for good speech recognition and sound quality across most environments. For children, it may be desirable to allocate frequencies out to at least 7,000 Hz. Children often require access to higher frequency speech inputs (i.e., >6,000 Hz) than adults in order to acquire optimal speech recognition and production (Stelmachowicz, Pittman, Hoover, & Lewis, 2001).

Input Dynamic Range (IDR)

As previously mentioned, the IDR parameter is implemented differently across the three cochlear implant systems; thus, device-specific management is discussed in Chapter 4. However, the lower end of the IDR functions similarly across the three manufacturers. The lower end of the IDR should correspond to an input level of approximately 25 dB SPL (i.e., average level for softest speech sounds) in the recipient's program for typical listening situations. The lower end of the IDR should never be increased for children. The pediatric population requires consistent access to soft speech to facilitate incidental learning, hear speech from a distance, and support optimal speech recognition. Adults may use a program in which the lower end of the IDR is elevated by 10 to 20 dB in order to improve speech understanding and comfort in noisy environments (i.e., restaurants). Also, when necessary, an increase in IDR of 5 to 10 dB may address complaints of low-level ambient noise in quiet environments.

Maxima

The maxima parameter is available only in *n*-of-*m* strategies. It determines how many channels will be stimulated at one time, and the channels selected are those with the greatest amplitudes. Preferred settings vary across individuals; however, research demonstrates that nine or more channels are required for optimal performance in noise (Dorman, Loizou, Spahr, & Maloff, 2002). In practice, the maxima parameter often is set between 10 and 12.

KEY CONCEPTS

The key information provided in this chapter should provide the reader a basic understanding of the following basic principles for cochlear implant programming:

■ Detailed counseling is necessary prior to cochlear implant activation to facilitate realistic expectations with the implant, discuss post-implant appointments, discuss typical performance at activation, and to review progression of typical improvements with the implant over time.

■ Following implantation, the recipient will receive a physical exam, imaging, and cochlear implant programming, which involves selection of a coding strategy, setting stimulation levels, and adjusting other parameters.

■ Several parameters that are available and adjustable on some cochlear implants systems include stimulation rate, pulse width, channel gain, frequency allocation, IDR, and maxima.

4

Manufacturer-Specific Programming Considerations

The three cochlear implant manufacturers in the United States each have developed sophisticated devices that allow many recipients with severe to profound hearing loss achieve remarkable open set speech recognition and communicative abilities. As discussed in Chapter 3, these systems share many similarities, but several differences exist in the hardware (Chapter 1), programming interface (i.e., connection to computer), computer software, clinician-adjustable parameters, signal coding strategies, and recommended programming protocols for sound processors in each system. The goal of this chapter is to provide detailed, device-specific information about programming of the most contemporary sound processors for each manufacturer. In addition, clinically relevant information will be provided for some of the earlier generation implants.

ADVANCED BIONICS CORPORATION

There are two different software platforms used to program Advanced Bionics implants. Recipients with the previous version C1 internal devices (i.e., C1.0 and C1.2) are programmed in the SCLIN software platform, and all users of the newer CII and 90K internal devices (i.e., 2001 to present) are programmed in the SoundWave software platform (version 1.4.77). The primary focus of this discussion will be on programming in SoundWave, but some general information will be provided on the SCLIN platform.

HiResolution (HiRes) 90K System

The most recent sound processor, the Harmony behind-the-ear (BTE), is compatible with the HiRes 90K or CII internal devices. People who use these internal implants also may use the Auria BTE or the Platinum Series body-worn sound processor. These processors are connected to the computer via an interface box referred to as the clinician's programming interface (CPI). The clinician must select either a specially designed BTE cable or a body-worn cable to couple the respective processor to the CPI. The programming platform provides the clinician with a simple and time-efficient system for determining appropriate program parameters for the HiRes cochlear implant signal coding strategies.

A series of color-coded icons reside in the lower right-hand corner of the SoundWave software.

These are used to inform the clinician of the status of the three primary components involved in the programming process: (1) the CPI, (2) the sound processor, and (3) the internal device. If the devices are all connected properly and identified by the programming computer, the icons are highlighted in green. Red highlighting indicates that the component is not detected by the computer, while yellow highlighting indicates the processor is connected, but is not ready for programming (e.g., an older processor not compatible with the SoundWave software, a faulty connection with a contemporary processor, etc.).

Electrode Impedance

When all three components are successfully identified by the programming computer, the software automatically measures electrode impedance at the 16 intracochlear electrode contacts relative to the case band reference electrode. Any impedance value between 1 and 30 killiohms is within normal limits. Results of all electrode impedance tests on the device are accessed through the Reports and Impedance History tabs. The impedance history report table also indicates explicitly any short or open electrode circuits. The clinician also may view impedance values in the programming screen. The clinician should disable these electrodes for the pediatric recipient's program. For adults, the clinician can ask the user to report whether sound quality and speech clarity is best supported by disabling both electrodes or leaving them enabled.

The clinician also may perform electrode conditioning to eliminate any substances present at the electrode contact (i.e., protein deposits, air bubbles) through the application of a low-level current. These unwanted substances typically cause elevated electrode impedances at initial activation of the implant; however, impedances almost always decrease over time with consistent stimulation.

Selecting a Signal Coding Strategy

The next step in programming is to select one of four signal coding strategies: HiRes-P (HiRes-Paired), HiRes-S (HiRes-Sequential), HiRes-P Fidelity 120, and HiRes-S Fidelity 120 (see Chapter 2 for descriptions of coding strategies). The authors recommend beginning with HiRes-S Fidelity 120 at initial activation with adults because the channel stimulation rate of 3712 pulses per second (pps) and per electrode stimulation rate of 1856 pps should be more than sufficient for most recipients. Furthermore, the sequential nature of electrode stimulation eliminates any chance for deleterious channel interaction, and the current steering across all electrodes may enhance the user's spectral resolution. Clinical trials with Fidelity 120 suggest that most users experience better sound quality for speech and music when compared to conventional HiRes sound processing (Advanced Bionics Corporation, 2009). Finally, the 18-microsecond pulse width should be more than sufficient to avoid voltage compliance issues for most recipients. As described in an upcoming section, the SoundWave software automatically manages the pulse width to avoid voltage compliance issues. At this time, the Fidelity 120 strategies have not received FDA approval for use with children.

Previous clinical trials show substantial variation in user preferences across the aforementioned signal coding strategies. For this reason, users should be given the opportunity to listen to each strategy, which is typically done at the one-week postactivation programming appointment. However, clinical judgment should be used to determine the appropriate time to introduce the different signal coding strategies. If the recipient is struggling to acclimate to the cochlear implant signal at the one-week appointment (i.e., difficulty tolerating sufficient stimulation, adjustment to sound quality, limited speech recognition capacity), the various signal coding strategies may be introduced at a later programming session.

Enhanced versions of the original Advanced Bionics signal coding strategies, Continuous Interleaved Sampling (CIS) and Multiple Pulsatile Sampler (MPS), also may be created in the SoundWave software platform. To create these strategies, the clinician will (1) open a HiRes-S (CIS) or HiRes-P (MPS) program, (2) disable all even-numbered electrodes, and (3) manually increase the pulse width to 75 microseconds. Most new recipients will be better served with one of the four default signal coding strategies; however, there are some experienced recipients who may prefer to remain with their older signal coding strategies. The reduced number of channels in the older signal coding strategies may limit channel interaction, which may be beneficial for a small subset of recipients. As mentioned in an earlier chapter, research suggests that recipients perform better with HiResolution sound processor than traditional coding strategies (Dunn, Tyler, Witt, & Gantz, 2006). One potential compromise to creating an older strategy is to leave all 16 electrode contacts active but change the pulse width to the same stimulation rate used for CIS or MPS. This compromise usually offers satisfactory sound quality for the user, and the additional channels will potentially enhance performance in noise.

Setting Stimulation Levels

In the SoundWave platform, stimulation levels are measured in charge units or clinical units. Charge units are the product of the amplitude of the stimulus current, the pulse width, and an arbitrary constant ($k = .013$). This unit of stimulation represents a constant charge, and its value is always the same, regardless of the pulse width. In other words, if the pulse width is increased, the current is decreased to maintain the same charge value. Specifically, when voltage compliance is reached, and increases in stimulus current amplitude can no longer be provided, the pulse width is automatically increased by the software. This frees the clinician from having to monitor the pulse width to ensure stimulation remains within voltage compliance. The range of stimulation levels provided by the software is 0 to 6000 charge units, but most M levels (i.e., upper stimulation levels) do not exceed 300 charge units. For more information for typical stimulation levels for children and adults in Advanced Bionics devices, the reader should refer to Zwolan and Overstreet (2005).

Clinicians also may increase manually the pulse width to a fixed level with the primary purpose of decreasing the stimulation rate. In fact, to adjust the stimulation rate in the SoundWave software, the clinician must adjust the pulse width. Changes to pulse width are also helpful if the clinician suspects that stimulation levels are approaching the maximum current limit because of voltage compliance restrictions. Higher current levels should be avoided because they increase the likelihood of channel interaction and nonauditory side effects, such as facial nerve stimulation.

In the default programming mode, the clinician is not required to measure T levels to create HiRes programs. Instead, the T level is automatically set to 10% of the established M-level value. In most cases, this estimation of T level allows recipients to access low-level sounds, and performance is similar between estimated and measured T levels. The clinician does, however, have the option to measure T levels manually or to set T levels to zero charge units. The only reason the latter option is performed is to eliminate complaints of constant, low-level noise that may arise from the continuous electrical stimulation or from the enhanced audibility of environmental sounds. Before any adjustments are made, the clinician should encourage the recipient to allow for a period of acclimatization. If the T levels are set to zero charge units, they can be adjusted at a later appointment to allow for access to low-level inputs.

T levels should be measured when the implant equipment (i.e., sound processor microphone, etc.) is functioning within normal limits and sound-field detection thresholds are elevated (i.e., child ≥25 dB HL; adult ≥30 dB HL). For adults, sound-field thresholds are more likely to be elevated when T levels are estimated and the recipient has a history of meningitis, long-term deafness, or abnormal cochlear anatomy. These conditions are all associated with spiral ganglion degeneration, which may result in a reduction in the user's electrical dynamic range. The clinician may consider measuring T levels for children because previous research emphasizes the importance of consistent audibility for young children. For measuring T levels in children, the authors suggest a 5-charge-unit-down and 10-charge-unit-up approach with tone-burst stimuli. Young children are likely to provide a minimal response level instead of a true threshold; therefore, after measuring T levels the clinician may consider a small global reduction (the authors use a 6 to 8 charge unit reduction) to lessen the possibility of child perceiving constant low-level electrical noise.

The default method of measuring M levels is unique in the Advanced Bionics programming platform. Instead of presenting biphasic pulses to individual electrode contacts, a Speech Burst stimulus is used. The Speech Burst consists of white noise filtered through three or four channels and is presented at the user's typical stimulation rate. There are three advantages to using Speech Burst stimuli over conventional programming stimuli. First, it more closely represents the spectral characteristics of complex speech and environmental sounds. Second, simultaneous presentation on multiple channels more closely resembles expected summation across channels in live speech mode and accounts for loudness summation (i.e., M levels may be more accurate). Third, simultaneous presentation across several channels is potentially more time efficient than single-channel measurements. Furthermore, Advanced Bionics' research studies show similar performance when using programs created using single-channel versus Speech Burst measures (Advanced Bionics, 2003).

In the default mode, clinicians should consider measuring M levels for each of the four Speech Burst bands (i.e., Speech 1–4, 5–8, 9–12, 13–16) in order to evaluate M levels across the electrode array. After these adjustments, the clinician may fine-tune the M levels globally while the recipient listens to live speech and environmental sounds. Once again, the M levels should be set to the point that is most comfortable for the recipient. Subsequently, loudness balancing procedures at M levels are recommended across two channels at a time. These measurements may be conducted in an apical to basal or basal to apical direction and are accomplished by manually presenting tone-burst stimuli on two neighboring channels in a sequential fashion. Typically, the task is easier for the recipient when three tone burst are presented on one channel followed by three tone bursts on the neighboring channel.

Furthermore, it should be noted that M levels also may be measured with single-channel tone-burst stimuli. Additionally, some clinicians choose to increase M levels globally (set at a flat profile) in live speech mode to the recipient's most comfortable listening level. Then, channel-specific (or band-specific) adjustments are made to address

sound quality complaints of the recipient or to improve speech clarity.

As mentioned in Chapter 3, upper stimulation levels are closely related to the electrically evoked stapedial reflex threshold (ESRT); therefore, this may be the ideal and most objective approach for setting M levels in many recipients (i.e., young children). The ESRT also is highly correlated to measured M levels when both were conducted with Speech Burst stimuli (Buckler & Overstreet, 2003). In addition, M levels based on Speech Burst ESRT may allow for better speech recognition than programs created via psychophysical loudness scaling (Wolfe & Kasulis, 2008). In many cases, recipients will prefer M levels that approach but do not reach their ESRT. To establish M levels based on ESRT, the clinician will (1) measure the ESRT across the electrode array (either with Speech Bursts or tone bursts), (2) decrease the M levels globally to a level that is soft to the recipient, (3) activate the sound processor in live speech mode, and (4) gradually increase M levels until the recipient indicates that the speech signal is most comfortable (see Chapter 3 for additional information). For children who are unable to provide verbal feedback about the signal, M levels should be set within 5 to 10% of their ESRT. For all recipients, it is unlikely that the M level will exceed the ESRT. In most cases, Speech Bursts are excellent stimuli for eliciting the ESRT; however, if the ESRT is variable and inconsistent in charge units across the electrode array (i.e., ESRT to Speech Burst for electrodes 9–12 is substantially higher than 13–16), then the clinician should consider measuring it with tone-burst stimuli.

Additional Programming Parameters

Microphone Sensitivity and Volume Control. The sensitivity of the Harmony and Auria sound processors can be adjusted in the SoundWave software, but typically, it should remain on the default setting. Essentially, the sensitivity controls the gain (+/–10 dB) applied to the signal as it is relayed from the microphone to the bandpass filters. Adjustments in sensitivity affect all frequencies equally. An increase in sensitivity will improve access to low-level sounds, but may degrade hearing in noisy environments. A decrease in microphone sensitivity may improve comfort in noise, but also will diminish audibility for low-level sounds (e.g., 20 to 25 dB SPL).

Adjustments to the volume control setting on any Advanced Bionics sound processor increases or decreases the stimulation provided at M level. The volume control parameter in SoundWave determines maximum and minimum M levels that may be obtained with changes to the volume control from the default setting (i.e., 12:00 on the processor). The extent to which the M level can be reduced ranges from 0 to +/−100% and is related to a percentage of the dynamic range. For instance, at a setting of −50%, reducing the volume control from the 12:00 position to the minimum position decreases the M level by 50% of the electrical dynamic range. For this example, if T level is 10 charge units and M level is 100 charge units, then adjusting the volume control from 12:00 to the minimum position will decrease the M level by 45 charge units [i.e., (100 − 10) * .5 = 45]. If the minimum setting is programmed to 0%, then a reduction in the volume control below the 12:00 position will not decrease the M level at all. This may be appealing for children who have no tolerance problems (i.e., tolerates M levels during all waking hours) and like to adjust their volume controls. Finally, if the lower end of the volume control is adjusted to −100%, reduction of the volume control to the minimum setting will result in M levels corresponding to T levels. When using this setting, low-level noise from the processor may not be audible. This may be appealing for new recipients who are acclimating to their implant or for children who prefer a low-level setting in the morning. In this case, adjustment from the minimum volume control setting to the preferred setting should typically take place over a few seconds.

The clinician should exercise caution when setting the upper range of the volume control parameter (i.e., +50%). In the aforementioned example, an upper-range value of 100% would allow the user to increase the M-level setting from 100 charge units at the 12:00 position to 190 charge units at the maximum position. If M levels are set accurately at the recommended user setting (i.e.,

12:00), then a 100-percent increase in stimulation relative to the electrical dynamic range (or even 50%) is rarely, if ever, appropriate. When the volume control provides too much latitude for increasing M levels, the user may encounter uncomfortable signal levels. As a result, for adults, the upper end of the volume control range should be set between 10 to 20% to allow a small increase in volume as needed. For children who have optionally programmed M levels (i.e., based on ESRT), the upper end of the volume control range should be set to 0 to prevent a further increase in M level stimulation and potential discomfort.

Channel Gains. As discussed in Chapter 3, the channel-gain parameter allows for frequency-specific adjustments to the gain of the signal from the microphone. As shown in Figure 4–1, channel gain may be adjusted in a broad manner by clicking on the channel gain Shape Icons in the SoundWave software or by accessing the channel-specific-gain values in the table located below the stimulation window (where T and M levels are adjusted). When a patient has appropriate stimulation levels, adjustment to channel gains may not be necessary. However, it may be helpful for recipients who cannot tolerate changes in M level and have complaints about sound quality. A program with reduced high-frequency channel gain could address issues with sound quality (e.g., too sharp/tinny) or discomfort, while reductions to low-frequency channel gains may improve listening comfort and performance in noisy environments. Increases to low-frequency gain channels will likely improve overall loudness, while increases to high-frequency gain channels may enhance sound quality.

Extended Filtering. Extended filtering will determine the lowest frequency represented in the low channel. In the default mode, Extended Low Filtering, the high-pass cutoff of channel 1 is set to 250 Hz with a center frequency of 333 Hz. In the Standard Filtering mode, the high-pass cutoff of channel 1 is increased to 350 Hz with a center frequency of 383 Hz. The vast majority of recipients will benefit from the extended low-frequency filtering. If an adult recipient complains of a pronounced

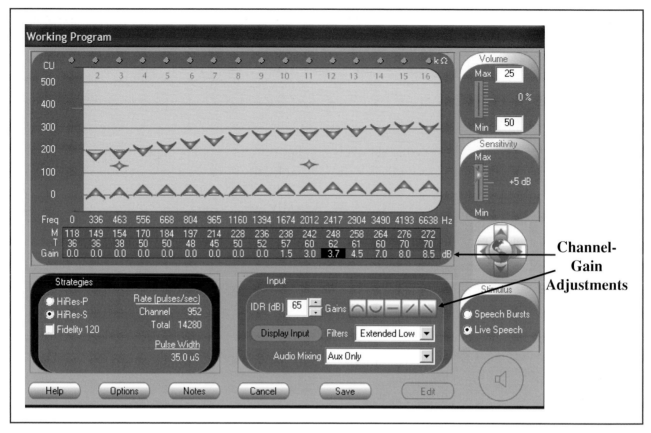

FIGURE 4–1. Channel-gain adjustment in the SoundWave software. Courtesy of Advanced Bionics (http://www.AdvancedBionics.com).

echo, intrusive ambient noise, or his or her own voice being too loud, it may be beneficial to try standard filtering.

Input Dynamic Range (IDR). In Advanced Bionics implants, the default IDR is 60 dB; therefore, inputs ranging from 25 to 85 dB SPL are mapped into the recipient's electrical dynamic range. Inputs below 25 dB SPL are discarded, and inputs exceeding 85 dB SPL are subjected to significant compression. Most recipients do very well with an IDR of 60 to 65 dB. Decreasing the IDR results in an increase in the "floor." For example, decreasing the IDR from 60 to 40 dB adjusts the acoustic inputs that are mapped to the lower end of the dynamic range from 25 to 45 dB (i.e., minimal influence to the upper end). At this modified setting, soft sounds will not be as audible, but listening comfort may be improved in noise. Increasing the IDR also influences inputs mapped

at the lower end of the dynamic range by positioning low-level sounds higher into the electrical dynamic range. In addition, the IDR increase will improve sound quality for high-level sounds and music appreciate by placing moderate to high-level sounds higher in the recipient's electrical dynamic range; thus, reducing the chances of high-level compression (Spahr, Dorman, & Loiselle, 2007). In fact, Advanced Bionics recommends creating a program with an increased IDR to enhance sound quality for music. The IDR can be adjusted from 20 to 80 dB and can be set on a program by program basis.

Audio-Mixing Ratio. The audio-mixing ratio adjusts the relative strengths of signals arriving from the microphone of the speech processor and an auxiliary source (e.g., FM system, iPod, T-Mic). A thorough discussion of audio-mixing settings and adjustments is provided in Chapter 7.

Lock. The HiRes 90K system possesses a unique feature called PoEM (Power Estimator) that is designed to optimize battery life as well as monitor and adjust the radio frequency (RF) power needed to maintain a consistent signal across a variety of listening environments. The system uses high RF levels only when absolutely necessary (i.e., high-level noise environments), and it automatically accounts for changes in skin-flap thickness that may occur over time. The PoEM also allows for use of the same program across multiple sound processors because the RF needs of each processor are determined during use, not during programming.

The PoEM mode can be disabled, and the clinician manually can adjust the RF level to a fixed setting. The need for a manual RF adjustment is a rare occurrence and is necessary only when the recipient reports signal intermittencies across various environments. In the Options menu, the clinician may access special PoEM parameters by simultaneously pressing the Ctrl+Shift+Alt+i keys. The programmer also may adjust the magnitude of the PoEM as well as the frequency in which the PoEM table is updated. PoEM's provision of a continuous estimation of power needs is attributed to the fact that the device uses two separate RF frequencies, one for forward telemetry (49 M Hz) and another (10.7 M Hz) for backward telemetry. This allows for a simultaneous exchange of information between the external and internal devices.

Automatic Gain Control (AGC). The AGC feature allows the clinician to disable the dual-action AGC, which is used to compress a wide range of signals within the IDR into the recipient's narrow electrical dynamic range. For the most part, this parameter should not be disabled because it allows recipients to perform well across a wide variety of environments (Spahr et al., 2007). However, the clinician may disable the AGC if the recipient complains that abrupt sounds or very loud sounds are "cut off" in environments with high-level noise.

Indifferent (Reference) Electrode Ground. When in the Options menu, the clinician also may push the ctrl+shift+alt+i keys to switch the reference electrode from the case band ground to the ring ground electrode located on the electrode lead. This is done only when the case band reference electrode is determined faulty or when significant facial nerve stimulation is present and cannot be resolved with other programming adjustments (i.e., increasing pulse width, channel clipping, or disabling one or more channels).

Channel Clipping. Channel clipping prevents stimulation from ever exceeding a predefined, fixed level. This is desirable when the user frequently adjusts the volume control, which results in adjustments to M levels. Clipping allows for an increase to stimulation on all channels except for the one in which clipping is implemented (clipping may be adjusted in a channel-by-channel basis). This is beneficial if stimulation at a certain level causes nonauditory side effects, such as facial nerve stimulation. In this case, clipping would be set at the highest stimulation level that does not provoke the undesired response.

Programming Previous Generations of Advanced Bionics Implants

All recipients with C1 and 1.2 internal devices are programmed in the SCLIN programming software. Many of the basic programming strategies used in SoundWave also are present in the SCLIN software. Therefore, clinicians who are familiar with SoundWave should easily adapt to SCLIN. There are, however, a few significant differences. First, SCLIN allows C1 and 1.2 devices to be programmed with the Simultaneous Analog Stimulation (SAS) signal coding strategy (see Chapter 2 for a description). An analog stimulus must be used to measure stimulation levels with the SAS strategy. The clinician will select either an analog stimulus or a train of biphasic pulses prior to making stimulation level measurements. Second, the clinician may select from three different types of AGC: AGC1, AGC2, or AGC off, and AGC2 is recommended for the vast majority of recipients. Third, at the end of the programming session, the clinician must use a special RF Power test to estimate the amount of RF power required to sufficiently operate the user's program with the sound processor. The test presents high-level environmental sounds (e.g., clapping) while the software estimates the optimal RF power necessary to provide efficient battery life and a consistent signal. Finally, the measurement of the electrically evoked compound action potential of the auditory nerve is not available for C1 devices, but is available via the Neural Response Imaging (NRI) platform in the SoundWave software.

COCHLEAR CORPORATION

At this time, the software platform used to program Cochlear Corporation Nucleus Freedom and CP810 sound processors, as well as older sound processors including ESPrit 3G and SPrint, is Custom Sound 3.0. This software provides a high level of control and flexibility to adjust parameters.

The Nucleus 5 System

The most recent sound processor of Cochlear Corporation is the CP810, which is part of the Cochlear Nucleus 5 system. The hardware used to connect the processor to the computer is shown in Figure 4–2. Briefly, a programming interface, known as a pod, is connected to the sound processor with specialized programming cable, and the pod is connected to the programming computer with a USB cable.

Electrode Impedance

The first step involved in programming in Custom Sound 3.0 is to measure electrode impedance in four different electrode coupling modes. The first mode, common ground, is the most sensitive for detecting anomalous intracochlear electrodes. Monopolar 1 and Monopolar 2 coupling modes identify the status of the remote reference electrode (located on the end of the nonstimulating electrode lead), respectively, via measurements of each intracochlear electrode. In the fourth mode, monopolar 1+2, each intracochlear electrode is referenced to the remote and case reference electrodes. This mode requires the lowest stimulation

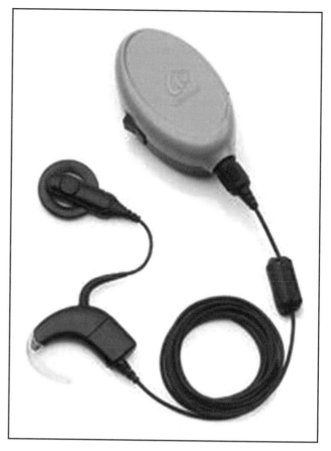

FIGURE 4–2. Programming pod and cable used to connect the Cochlear Americas Nucleus CP810 Sound Processor to the computer. Courtesy of Cochlear™ Americas, © 2009 Cochlear Ltd.

levels, provides the highest consistency in stimulation needs across the electrode array, and reflects the typical impedance of stimulation used on a daily basis.

Electrode impedances below 565 ohms are abnormal and designated as "short" circuits, and electrode impedances greater than 30 kohms are abnormally high and are referred to as "open" circuits. Electrodes with abnormal impedances are disabled (i.e., flagged) and deactivated for programming and subsequent impedance assessments. At initial activation, impedance is frequently high but will generally decrease with routine implant use. Therefore, the clinician should reassess impedance at later appointments to monitor electrode status. The clinician may re-activate any flagged electrodes in the Recipient/Edit menu in the software. This will allow for reassessment and subsequent determination of availability for programming in the patient's MAP. Short-circuited electrodes are often permanently faulty because of compromised contacts or leads and should not be activated in recipient programs due to the possibility of poor sound quality and performance.

Selecting a Signal Coding Strategy and Preprocessing Parameters

The next step involved in programming in Custom Sound 3.0 is to select a signal coding strategy, stimulation rate, maxima, and other processing parameters. The ACE signal coding strategy is recommended initially because previous clinical trials show that it provides superior average performance over CIS and SPEAK strategies (Beynon, Snik, & van den Broek, 2003; Manrique et al., 2005; Skinner et al., 2002). Moreover, previous research suggests that subjects have optimal speech-recognition performance when using a stimulation rate of 900 pps or greater and at least 9 maxima (Balkany et al., 2007; Dorman, Loizou, Spahr, & Maloff, 2002). That authors recommend beginning with 11 maxima to provide sufficient detail for a speech signal embedded in competing noise and, with that number of maxima, the widest pulse width possible is 37 microseconds/phase. A wider pulse width requires less current level for a given psychophysical percept, which may reduce the potential for deleterious channel interaction. Skinner, Holden, and Holden (1994, 1997) have shown that narrow frequency allocation in the midfrequency channels results in better speech recognition. With that in mind, the authors also recommend setting the frequency allocation table's upper boundary out to approximately 7,000 Hz for children and 6,000 to 6,500 Hz for adults. All other processing parameters should remain at default settings for the initial program. If the recipient is not making satisfactory progress after six months of implant use, the clinician may try alternative signal coding strategies or stimulation rates (see Chapter 3). It also should be noted that most recipients will experience satisfactory outcomes when the signal coding parameters are set to the default settings. The authors use the aforementioned recommendations, which have been

successful with recipients. Additional parameters for adjustment are discussed later in this chapter, but the reader should keep in mind that in many cases, adjustments to these parameters are not necessary. Again, the provision of appropriate T and C levels is the most important factor that influences recipient success.

Setting Stimulation Levels

When creating a new program in Custom Sound 3.0, five channels (22, 16, 11, 6, and 1) are highlighted for measurement. The streamlined approach to programming suggests that the clinician measure stimulation levels on these five channels and interpolate the remaining values. This procedure is supported by research, which shows equivalent performance for programs created with the streamlined and conventional approaches (Plant et al., 2005). However, to detect any potential variation across the array, the authors also recommend measuring stimulation levels on at least one channel between each of these five highlighted channels as well as channels 2 and 3. At the following appointment, the clinician should attempt to measure stimulation levels across a variety of channels; conversely, in young children, stimulation levels should be measured on as many channels possible.

As discussed in Chapters 2 and 3, the measurement of accurate T and C levels is crucial in providing a high-quality program. For the Nucleus 5 system, the T level is the lowest level of stimulation that the user can detect 100% of the time. Appropriate alternatives for measuring T levels were discussed in Chapter 3, but typically, The authors of this book use a clinical-bracketing approach with two stimulus presentations at each current level (CL). At initial stimulation, a 5 CL ascending step size and a 10 CL descending step size is used. For experienced adults and attentive children, ascending and descending step sizes are set to 2 and 4 CL, respectively. Increases in CL occur logarithmically and range from 0 CL (10 microamperes) to 255 CL (1.75 milliamperes) at a given pulse width. The pulse width may vary from 9 to 400 microseconds/phase.

When T levels are set too high, the user may complain of ongoing noise. To determine whether this complaint of noise is from elevated T levels or normal ambient noise, the clinician can increase the floor of the IIDR by increasing the T-SPL parameter or decreasing the sensitivity. If the unwanted perception persists, T levels should be decreased globally. However, if it is diminished, the user should be encouraged to adapt to the normal ambient noise.

The upper stimulation levels, C levels, should be perceived by the user as "loud but comfortable." Approaches to measuring C levels were discussed in Chapter 3, but briefly, C levels should be set initially using the ESRT and then adjusted to a comfortable level in live speech mode. Typically, optimal performance and sound quality are achieved when C levels are 10 to 20 CL below the ESRT values. When C levels are more than 20 CL below the ESRT for experienced CI users (>3 months), the clinician should gradually increase stimulation levels until they are within 15 CL of the ESRT. On the other hand, if C levels exceed the ESRT, the clinician should counsel the recipient to accept a lower-stimulation setting that is within 5-CL of the ESRT. In most cases, once the recipient has time to adjust to the lower ESRT-based C levels, performance will improve. In addition, setting C levels above ESRT may lead to constant stapedial reflex contraction during regular implant use, which is atypical for the auditory system.

If the ESRT cannot be measured, the clinician may use psychophysical loudness scaling to set C levels to a "loud but comfortable" percept in each channel across the electrode array. Finally, when setting C levels globally in live speech mode, a small step size of 2 CL may be used to adjust the C levels to the "loud but comfortable" percept. Increases in stimulation in the Custom Sound 3.0 software occur in a logarithmic fashion and may cause loudness growth with small changes to C levels. After these global adjustments, small increases (e.g., 2 CL) may slightly improve clarity and sound quality, but should be made only when the recipient will tolerate the increased loudness. The clinician should continue to make 2-CL increases until the user reports distortion or discomfort. At this point, a 3- to 4-CL decrease often will be ideal for the user.

When ESRT cannot be measured, another alternative is to (1) superimpose C levels at the measured T levels and (2) adjust C levels globally in live speech mode to a level that is "loud but comfortable." This approach results in an electrical dynamic range that is equal across the electrode array, but should be used a last resort because T- and C-level configurations often differ.

Additional Programming Parameters

Input Processing. The next step in CustomSound 3.0 is to consider using the input preprocessing characteristics (i.e., SmartSound processing), which include Autosensitivity, Adaptive Dynamic Range Optimization (ADRO), and Beam (multimicrophone directionality). Based on previous research, optimal speech recognition of low-level inputs (James et al., 2002; Müller-Deile, Kiefer, Wyss, Nicolai, Battmer, 2008) and in noisy environments (Wolfe et al., 2009) should be achieved when using ADRO and Autosensitivity, respectively. Therefore, the Autosensitivity+ADRO setting should be selected as the recipient's primary program in the Write to Processor screen where new programs are loaded into the sound processor. The specific characteristics of the input preprocessing in the Nucleus 5 system is described in detail later in this chapter.

Microphone Sensitivity and Volume Control. In Custom Sound 3.0, the clinician may program the CP810 sound processor in a simple or advanced mode. In the simple mode, the user must access volume and sensitivity setting adjustments via the CR110 wireless remote assistant. In the advanced mode, the recipient may adjust volume or sensitivity with the buttons on the processor by selecting the Advanced (volume) or Advanced (sensitivity) mode, respectively, in the Processor Configuration menu.

A microphone sensitivity of 12 should be used by adults and children in most situations. Children should have a fixed sensitivity setting with Autosensitivity (i.e., automatic adjustments to sensitivity) engaged. Adults also may use Autosensitivity, or when appropriate, they may use the CR110 wireless remote control to change sensitivity settings. Example situations in which recipients report that manual adjustment may be helpful include (1) when speech and noise are too soft with Autosensitivity responding to background noise, (2) when better access to sounds originating from a distance (e.g., nature sounds when on a walk) is desired, and (3) when they wish to provide even further decreases in sensitivity to competing noise in an environment with high-level ambient noise.

Parents are still able to adjust the volume setting via the CR110 wireless assistant; however, these changes must be warranted to justify alteration to the child's carefully programmed C levels. The volume control also may be disabled for young children who have stable program levels. This may be accomplished by setting the volume-control range to 0% in the Parameters section of the Set Levels screen. It is likely that future versions of the Custom Sound software will allow the clinician to lock the sensitivity settings of the processor. There are, however, older children will desire to access the volume control. The volume control buttons of the CP810 can be locked on the processor and with the CR110 wireless assistant, and the volume control buttons of the CR110 also may be locked.

Adults often prefer to have access to their volume controls, which allows for adjustments across 10 steps (1–10). The range in which the volume control adjusts C levels is from 0 to 100% and is controlled by the "Volume Adjustment (%DR)" parameter. When the volume parameter is left at the default setting of 20%, decreasing the volume control from the maximum (i.e., 10) to the minimum (i.e., 1) results in a global reduction in C levels that corresponds to 20% of the recipient's electrical dynamic range. Therefore, a participant with an electrical dynamic range of 30 CL would experience a 6 CL decrease in stimulation when adjusting the volume control from 10 to 1 (30 CL * 20% = 6 CL). Small volume-adjustment settings (i.e., 30% or less of DR) allow for more precise control over the C level. Large changes to volume settings should not be necessary as long as C levels are set appropriately. However, broader control over the C levels may be helpful to new implant users, particularly when they first put the processor on in the morning.

At initial activation, allow the recipient or caregiver to adjust the volume down by 80 to 100% of their dynamic range. Parents are advised to start with the volume setting of 0 when the child first wakes up from sleep. The external transmitting coil should then be placed on the child's head and the volume of the processor should be increased to the desired setting (typically 8–10) over the next few seconds. If the child reacts negatively to the signal, the volume control should be adjusted to a comfortable setting, and the parent should attempt to increase the volume at a later point in the morning. If the child shows no reaction, the next time the processor is placed on the child's head, the parent should begin at a volume setting of approximately 2 to 3 and gradually increase the starting volume setting over the next few days or weeks. Once the recipient is able to tolerate the program with the volume control at a stable position, the range of the Volume Adjustment parameter should be decreased or the control should be disabled. For adults, the C levels are adjusted to provide a most comfortable loudness percept with the volume control set at a setting of 7 or 8, which allows the user to adjust the volume upward or downward from the recommended setting established during programming. For young children, comfortable upper stimulation levels are set with the volume control at the maximum setting (e.g., 10) to prevent increases in the volume control and a potentially uncomfortable loudness percept.

Adults and older children should understand the functions of the sensitivity and volume parameters to enable them to address listening difficulties. Sensitivity influences the audibility of soft sounds and compression of loud sounds, while the volume control adjusts the C levels up or down. Therefore, if patients feel that a listening environment is too soft or loud, they can adjust the volume control up or down, respectively. However, if soft sounds from a distance are inaudible, especially in quiet situations, they can increase the sensitivity. Understanding the function of these parameters will give experienced users the ability to address several common difficulties in quiet and noisy listening situations. It should be noted that when Autosensitivity is used, there is essentially no need to adjust the sensitivity setting manually. With Autosensitivity, most users are best served by adjusting the volume control instead. Also, in the CP810, the sensitivity parameter affects the strength of the signal delivered from the sound processor microphone as well as the accessory or telecoil signal. For all earlier generation processors, the sensitivity adjustment affects only the strength of the signal from the microphone.

T-SPL, C-SPL, and the IIDR. The instantaneous input dynamic range (IIDR) is a parameter label that is specific to Cochlear Ltd. implants and determines the range of acoustic inputs that are coded by the sound processor at any one point in time. The default IIDR of the Nucleus 5 and Freedom cochlear implants is 40 dB in order to capture the range of ongoing speech, from peaks to valleys, at a given input level. The T-SPL and C-SPL parameters adjust the lower and upper ends of the IIDR, respectively. A default T-SPL setting of 25 dB SPL suggests that inputs at 25 dB correspond to T levels, while below and above 25 dB are mapped below and above T levels, respectively. The default setting for the C-SPL is 65 dB SPL. This refers to the fact that, at a microphone setting of 12, inputs exceeding 65 dB SPL are subjected to infinite compression. The aforementioned intensity may be associated with loud speech and speech in noisy environments; therefore, sensitivity adjustments via manual or automatic (i.e., Autosensitivity) changes are critical. As shown in Figure 2–5, an adjustment of the sensitivity control allows for the IIDR window to be positioned at various input levels. Thus, the IDR, or the total range of input levels the processor can encode without significant clipping or distortion, is much wider than the IIDR. Wolfe et al. (2009) showed that activation of Autosensitivity was necessary to allow for adequate speech recognition in noise across a wide range of ambient noise levels. As a result, the clinician should consider engaging Autosensitivity for the recipient's primary program to be used in most typical listening situations.

As long as the clinician counsels patients to allow for an adjustment period to new sounds, adjustments to T-SPL and C-SPL parameters are rarely needed. When adults cannot acclimate to hearing low-level ambient noise (e.g., ventilation systems), the T-SPL parameter may be slightly increased; however, it should never be increased for young children. Adjustments to C-SPL are not desired because decreases will result in compression of everyday inputs and increases will make conversational speech too soft.

Autosensitivity Breakpoint. As previously mentioned, Autosensitivity (ASC) is a special type of input preprocessing exclusive to the Cochlear Ltd. SmartSound programming platform. The goal of ASC is to ensure that speech is always positioned 15 dB above background noise via automatic adjustments to the microphone sensitivity. In quiet environments, ASC is not operational. However, when the noise exceeds the default ASC breakpoint setting of 57 dB SPL, the digital ASC algorithm is engaged. It continuously analyzes the intensity of the competing noise during pauses in speech to determine the sensitivity reduction necessary to preserve the +15 dB speech-to-noise ratio. The reduction in microphone sensitivity prevents the peaks of speech from being embedded within the background noise. Previous research suggests that use of ASC significantly improves speech recognition in noise relative to performance with fixed sensitivity settings (Wolfe et al., 2009).

The ASC breakpoint may be adjusted in the Environment Configuration menu in the Write to Processor screen. It may be decreased down to 45 dB SPL when the recipient complains that background noise is still too loud and bothersome after ASC has engaged. In contrast, it may be increased up to 65 dB SPL if the recipient complains that speech and noise are too soft when ASC is activated. In our experience, the ASC breakpoint rarely needs to be adjusted, but future research is needed to determine how it might be optimized for each individual.

Loudness Growth. The loudness growth parameter determines the steepness of the logarithmic function used to map input sounds into the recipient's electrical dynamic range. This parameter rarely, if ever, should be adjusted. The loudness growth default setting is 20. Decreases and increases to loudness growth result in the mapping of inputs at higher or lower levels in the user's electrical dynamic range.

Jitter. The jitter parameter is available only for the SPEAK signal coding strategy. At low, fixed stimulation rates (e.g., 250 pps or lower), the recipient could perceive a continuous, low-pitched tonal sound that corresponds to the frequency of the stimulation rate. In essence, the auditory nerve is responding in a phase-locked manner to multiples of the stimulus rate, which is a normal auditory-system function for pitch coding. Jitter causes the stimulation rate to vary randomly by a certain percentage (e.g., 10%) around the stimulation rate. This random variation around the dominant stimulation rate eliminates the user's perception of a continuous low-pitched sound.

Telecoil-Mixing Ratio. The telecoil-mixing ratio determines the relative strength of signals from the telecoil and the sound processor microphone. The processor's built-in telecoil receives signals via electromagnetic induction and may be activated manually or in automatic mode for hearing on telecoil compatible telephones or in conjunction with hearing-assistance technology (e.g., FM system with neckloop). The different telecoil-mixing ratios and assistive device options will be discussed in Chapter 7. In Custom Sound 3.0, the default Telecoil-Mix ratio is 3:1, but the user may adjust the ratio with the CR110 wireless remote control to allow for more or less emphasis from the sound processor microphone. For the Freedom sound processor, the fixed telecoil-mixing ratio must be adjusted by the clinician in the software. If multiple Telecoil-Mix ratios are desired, the clinician must create a different program for each ratio.

Accessory-Mixing Ratio. The accessory-mixing ratio functions exactly the same as the telecoil-mixing ratio, but it influences the relative strength of signals from the sound processor microphone and the direct audio input source. In addition, when an accessory source (e.g., FM receiver, MP3 player) is plugged into the processor, the floor of the IIDR is automatically attenuated by 10 dB, even when set to 1:1. Also, with the Freedom processor and all predecessors, adjustments to the microphone sensitivity parameter through manual adjustments via ASC affect the strength of the signal from the sound processor microphone, but not the signal from the accessory source. However, with the CP810, an adjustment to the sensitivity setting affects the strength of the signal from both the sound processor microphone

and the accessory source. As a result, the clinician must recommend a higher mixing ratio rather than a sensitivity adjustment to achieve an "accessory advantage." The default accessory-mixing ratio is 2:1 (i.e., 6 dB reduction to processor microphone), but there are several other ratios that are discussed in Chapter 7. In addition to changes in the software, adjustments to mixing ratios also may occur via the CR110 wireless remote assistant.

Channel Gains. Channel gains allow for frequency-specific adjustments of +10.5 dB/−12 dB to the input signal from the sound processor microphone. When using ACE, changes to channel gain will influence whether or not the channel will be selected as a maxima because the gain adjustment is implemented at the input before the signal is processed. Because high frequencies contribute greatly to speech clarity, it is not desirable to reduce the gain for high-frequency channels. As a result, adjustment of channel gains in n-of-m strategies, such as ACE, should be avoided. Adjustments to stimulation levels to address sound quality issues would be preferred.

Voltage Compliance. Voltage compliance levels can be measured in Custom Sound 3.0. These levels indicate the maximum stimulus current amplitude, which is limited by the voltage capacity and the power source. For the Nucleus 5 system, Cochlear recommends that five or fewer channels are outside of voltage compliance limits by less than 10% on each channel. If these criteria are not met, the recipient will likely experience poor performance and sound quality because the loudness relationships across the channels will be compromised. Also, use of maximum current levels increases the likelihood of channel interaction and decreases battery life.

Voltage compliance issues should be easy to address through programming adjustments. Specifically, the clinician should increase the pulse width of the compromised channel and re-measure T and C levels. The increase in pulse width should decrease the current required to elicit a desired loudness percept. Voltage compliance problems were frequently encountered when using the Nucleus Freedom sound processor with the two-zinc-air mini controller as the power source.

However, the transmitting properties of the CP810 are more efficient, and the programs of most all recipients can be supported by a two-zinc-air battery pack.

Prediction of Stimulation Levels from Other Programs. In Custom Sound 3.0, the question mark icon can be used to estimate stimulation levels based on measured T and C levels in another program. Once a program is complete, the clinician can begin a new program with the same signal coding strategy but a different stimulation rate. The T and C levels are then measured for one channel, and the remaining channels can be predicted by clicking on the question mark icon. This feature allows for efficient creation of several programs with varying stimulation rates, which will aid the user in determining the optimal rate for long-term use.

Power Level. The power level determines the strength of the RF signal necessary from the external transmitting coil to the internal device without corruption of the original signal. The power level is automatically estimated in Custom Sound 3.0 when voltage compliance levels are measured and when new programs are loaded onto the sound processor. Power level is determined by stimulation levels, electrode impedance, and skin flap thickness, and it should be measured at every programming session. The automatic power level estimate is sufficient for the vast majority of recipients. However, if the recipient complains that the signal "cuts out" in noisy environments, the clinician may want to set manually the RF power level to 10% higher than the estimated value.

A power level of 100% corresponds to the maximum voltage the processor can provide. Each sound processor and battery option possess a theoretical power level maximum limit. For instance, with the Freedom sound processor, a power level of 56% is the maximum RF power level that can be supported by the mini, two-zinc-air controller. The maximum RF power level supported by the three-zinc-air battery controller is 75%, and the body-worn, two-AAA-alkaline battery controller provides the highest power-level capacity. The CP810 sound processor and cable/coil are more efficient than the Freedom sound processor and

cable/coil, and as a result, the maximum power level limit for the CP810 two-zinc-air battery case is much greater than that of the Freedom. However, because the maximum power level is determined on a processor-specific basis, it is not appropriate to compare Freedom power level to the CP810 power level. With that said, the maximum power level supported by the two-battery module of the CP810 is 77%, while the rechargeable batteries (not yet approved for clinical use by the United States Food and Drug Administration) are associated with a 100-percent power level. Given the power constraints of the different processors, explicit instructions are provided as to which battery options are suitable for use by a recipient. In most cases, all battery options are suitable, but in some rare cases, the mini-sized battery options may not provide sufficient power toward the end of the battery life. Because children may not be able to report potential sound quality issues, they should use battery options that will guarantee suitable power.

It is important to note that the power-level estimation is sometimes inaccurate for recipients with very thin skin flaps. These cases are identified by alerts from the programming software. In this occurs, the clinician may adhere a layer of mole skin to the underneath side of the coil or use a small plastic ring (spacer) provided by Cochlear to attach to the underneath side of the coil. Either solution artificially increases the width of the skin flap.

SmartSound Preprocessing. As mentioned earlier in this chapter, the Nucleus system offers several SmartSound preprocessing strategies that are designed to enhance listening abilities in a variety of situations. These strategies include ADRO, ASC, Beam, and Whisper. Of these strategies, ADRO and ASC are the most relevant and important for everyday use.

The objective of ADRO is to improve audibility for low-level sounds, maintain comfort for high-level inputs, and optimize the wide range of speech inputs into the user's narrow electrical dynamic range. This is accomplished by adaptively adjusting the channel gains based on the spectral characteristics, intensity, and ratio of the incoming speech and noise in the environment. Research demonstrates that ADRO significantly improves the recognition of soft speech in quiet and does not degrade performance in noise (Dawson, Decker, & Psarros, 2004; James et al., 2002). As a result, ADRO preprocessing should be enabled in all programs. Use of ADRO may initially result in a signal that is perceived as "too loud." If this occurs, C levels should be decreased slightly by 2 to 3 CL.

ASC was discussed in a previous section. ASC does not affect speech recognition in quiet as it automatically disengages in quiet settings, and it significantly improves speech recognition in noise (Wolfe et al., 2009). As a result, ASC should be used in conjunction with ADRO for the vast majority of listening environments.

Beam preprocessing, also referred to as Focus SmartSound preprocessing, utilizes the outputs of both processor microphones to create an adaptively varying directional microphone response. In noisy environments, the nulls of the Focus directional pattern are positioned to provide maximum attenuation of the competing noise. However, this adaptive attenuation is disengaged when speech is present in the rear hemisphere. The focus mode significantly improves speech recognition in noise when speech is presented in front of the listener and the noise is from the side and back (Spriet et al., 2007). Focus should be used by adults in conjunction with ADRO and ASC, but only in noisy environments where the primary talker will be in front of the user. In addition, the recipient must be counseled to face the talker and maintain a close proximity (i.e., 4 feet).

The goal of Whisper is to enhance audibility for low-level signals that originate from a distance. At default settings, the Freedom and CP810 sound processors provide audibility for inputs down to 25 dB SPL. In addition, ADRO enhances access to these low-level sounds. As a result, Whisper is not as critical for accessing soft sounds. However, it does place low-to-moderate level sounds (e.g., ≤52 dB SPL) into a higher position in the electrical dynamic range relative to typical settings. This may be helpful for stimuli with a wide range of inputs, such as music, but may impair speech recognition in noise. Therefore, the authors do not recommend routine use of Whisper for listening to speech. Nevertheless, it may be a good option for recipients who are able to activate it when listening to music.

SmartSound Environment Personalization. In Custom Sound 3.0, multiple programs or "overlays" to MAPs can be provided in the Write to Processor screen. These programs may vary in stimulation levels or preprocessing features. For example, they may have successively higher C levels to allow a new recipient to acclimate gradually to higher levels of stimulation. Once stimulation levels are appropriate, programs will have identical stimulation levels but may provide different types of SmartSound preprocessing. At this time, Cochlear recommends four programs with distinctive combinations of SmartSound: (1) Every day: ADRO + Autosensitivity, (2) Noise: ADRO + Autosensitivity (clinician may lower the Breakpoint of Autosensitivity to make more aggressive), (3) Focus: ADRO + ASC + Beam, and (4) Music: ADRO + Whisper. The different variations of SmartSound preprocessing with the same MAP are referred to as overlays.

Indicators. A variety of indicators may be selected in the Processor Configuration menu. First, a private alarm, audible only to the user, will indicate program changes and battery life. An audible public alarm presented through the CR110 remote assistant is also available, which can be enabled and disabled via the remote assistant. Second, there is an optional LED light that indicates the status of the processor and the program in use; the LED light also can be deactivated with the remote control.

Automatic Telecoil. As mentioned previously, the CP810 has an automatic telecoil that engages when a fluctuating electromagnetic signal with desirable speech-like characteristics is present from a nearby telephone or induction loop system. When the Auto Telecoil is enabled in the Custom Sound 3.0 software, the user may enable or disable the automatic telecoil feature with the CR110 remote assistant; however, when this feature is disabled in the software, it is unavailable to the user even via the remote control. In this case, the user manually can engage and disengage the telecoil with the CR110 remote assistant and with a button located on the upper spine of the processor. There is no remote assistant for the Freedom sound processor; therefore, the indicators selected by the clinician are fixed for each program. In addition, the audible public alarm is available only within the Freedom body-worn configuration.

Double Channel Mapping. The Custom Sound 3.0 programming software also allows double channel mapping. This mapping involves directing the outputs of two channels into one intracochlear electrode contact, which may be desirable when the recipient has a restricted number of channels due to disabled electrodes. When patients have restricted channels, the range of input frequencies is limited (i.e., 5500 versus 7000 Hz). Double channel mapping results in an increased bandwidth assigned to each electrode contact and an increased overall bandwidth for the recipient.

Channel-to-Electrode Assignment. At default settings, the Cochlear system allocates 22 channels to the 22 active intracochlear electrode contacts. Electrode 1 (and channel 1) is assigned to the most basal contact, and the electrode contact/channel number becomes progressively higher toward the apical end of the cochlea. The audiologist can reassign a channel to a different electrode contact by clicking on the active electrode coordinate within the Parameters Table and selecting the desired allocation. This procedure may be warranted on two rare occasions. First, it may be beneficial for recipients who do not have the expected tonotopic organization as determined by sweeping the programming stimulus across the electrode array. In this case, alterations are made to the channel-to-electrode assignment with the intention of restoring tonotopic organization. Second, if the recipient has a common cavity cochlea, the surgeon may choose to insert the electrode array through a cochleostomy made near the horizontal semicircular canal (i.e., opposite the typical direction). This procedure requires the clinician to invert the channel-to-electrode assignment, which places the higher-numbered electrodes at the basal end of the cochlea and the lower-numbered electrodes at the apical end.

Bilateral Mapping. The Custom Sound 3.0 platform allows for simultaneous mapping of recipients with bilateral cochlear implants via two programming pod interfaces connected to the computer.

The Bilateral Balancing tab allows for the activation of the bilateral sound processors in live speech mode. Global adjustments to T and C levels will ensure loudness balance between the two ears for speech and environmental sounds. Most users require a slight individualized reduction in C levels when listening in the bilateral mode compared to the unilateral conditions, which is likely related to binaural summation.

Programming Previous Generations of Nucleus Implants

Cochlear Ltd. has made a conscientious effort to offer the latest sound processor technology to its earliest recipients (Nucleus 22 users). In addition, the same programming software can be used across all generations of implants, which greatly simplifies programming for clinicians. The basic principles described in the previous section will enable a clinician to program most Nucleus implants with a few exceptions. First, Nucleus 22 internal devices must use the SPEAK signal coding strategy, which requires bipolar (BP) electrode coupling (see Chapter 2). The current default electrode coupling mode is BP+3 where the reference electrode is four electrodes apical to the stimulating electrode (however, when the SPEAK was first introduced, the default mode was BP+1, and many users continue to use that today). As a result, the four most apical electrodes are disabled in the user's program. If adequate loudness growth cannot be achieved with this configuration, a wider bipolar coupling mode (e.g., BP+4) may be used. Finally, a "variable" electrode coupling mode in SPEAK allows the clinician to vary the bipolar coupling mode (i.e., BP+1, BP+2, BP+3, etc.) from one electrode to the next. In the variable mode, the clinician should ensure that the expected tonotopic organization exists by sweeping at C level from apex to base.

Secondly, the Nucleus 22 device and the ESPrit 3G external sound processor are not capable of making telemetry measures. As a result, the RF power required to provide a signal with consistent integrity across a variety of environments will need to be measured. Also, the clinician should perform a Skin Flap measure to estimate its thickness (i.e., density). This information is used to estimate and optimize the RF power used in the recipient's program. For the ESPrit 3G device, the clinician also must perform a Power Optimization Test to estimate the necessary RF power level.

Finally, stimulation levels in the Nucleus 22 device may be measured in Stimulus Level units or Current Level units, the same scale used for contemporary devices. When using Current Level units, the pulse width is set at a fixed value. However, with Stimulus Level units, the pulse amplitude and the pulse width change in a complex manner to provide the shortest possible pulse width. As a result, Stimulus Level units are preferred, but Current Level units may be used if manual determination of the pulse width is potentially advantageous.

MED-EL CORPORATION

There are two programming platforms for MED-EL cochlear implants. The CI.STUDIO+ platform is used for recipients with TEMPO+ BTE and CISPRO+ body-worn sound processors, and the MAESTRO software platform is used for the more recent OPUS 1 and OPUS 2 sound processors. Recipients with the COMBI 40+, $PULSAR_{CI}^{100}$, and $SONATA_{TI}^{100}$ internal devices can all be programmed in the MAESTRO software as long as they use the OPUS 1 or OPUS 2 sound processors. The primary focus of this discussion will be on programming in MAESTRO, but general information will be provided on CI.STUDIO+.

Programming MED-EL Recipients in Fine Structure Processing

The most recent sound processor from MED-EL, the OPUS 2 BTE, may be used with any internal MED-EL device available in the USA. The processor is connected to the programming computer via the Diagnostic Interface Box II (DIB II), which has two color-coded ports for various MED-EL sound processors and a port for the DIB coil, which is used for telemetry and ART measure-

ments. The green port is used for the CISPRO+ body-worn processors (almost obsolete), the blue port is used for all BTE processors, and the yellow port is used for telemetry measures (i.e., electrode impedance). The yellow port also is used for assessment of the electrical compound action potential (ECAP) in the Auditory Response Telemetry (ART) platform and to identify characteristics specific to the user's internal device (i.e., serial number, voltage distribution in the cochlea). The MAESTRO software platform is designed to provide a simple and rapid approach for establishing recipient programs.

Electrode Impedance

The first step in creating a Fine Structured Processing (FSP) program is to measure impedance at the 12 intracochlear electrode contacts relative to the reference electrode in the Impedance Field Telemetry (IFT) section of the MAESTRO software. The IFT task also allows for measures of voltage distribution across all intracochlear electrodes when one active electrode is stimulated. Impedance results of the 12 intracochlear and one reference electrodes are displayed in kilohms in the IFT table. The software indicates an electrical impedance that is abnormal by noting a "greater than" (>) sign next to the impedance value, or, in the case of an open circuit, by listing the channel status as "HI." The impedance of the reference electrode is affected by the surrounding tissue, the current conduction through the extracochlear medium, and the mechanical status of the electrode. The status of each electrode is provided under the impedance value and includes one of the following five categories. First, the *"OK"* status suggests that the voltage is within normal limits and suitable for stimulation. Second, the *"HI"* status indicates that the voltage exceeds the limits of the system and cannot provide sufficient current flow. These channels should be deactivated. Third, the *"SC-x"* status refers to a short circuit and indicates that the signal also is traveling to another intracochlear electrode. The letter following the "SC" allows the clinician to identify which channels are shorted together in the event that more than one short circuit is present. Electrodes with short circuits should be disabled.

Fourth, the "*SC?*" status indicates the rare situation where the software was unable to determine the channel status and is intended to cue the clinician to check the voltage table f manually or a possible short. Electrode shorts can be manually identified by reviewing the "Voltage Distribution Profile" table, which is described in the next section. Fifth, the "*HSC-x*" status suggests abnormally high electrode impedance in addition to electrical coupling to another electrode. The result of test is generally intended to identify possible short circuits when the implant is tested in its sterile packaging, prior to implantation; it identifies possible short circuits even in the presence of very high impedance on the channels (as would be expected when the electrode and ground contacts are not contacting fluid or tissue). If the voltage table confirms the presence of a short circuit, both electrode contacts should be disabled. However, if additional shorts are identified, the clinician should contact the MED-EL representative. A "HSC?" status is shown when the reference electrode impedance is not measured correctly (although this is a rare finding when measured in vivo). Again, the VDP table will aid the clinician with electrode management.

In addition to the impedance value and status, the table also displays the serial number of the internal SONATA$_{TI}$^{100}and PULSAR$_{CI}$^{100} devices and the total number of functional, shorted, and open electrodes. Furthermore, the table describes the "integrity of the internal device electronics" and the quality of the coupling between the DIB II coil and the internal device. On the Integrity test, an "OK" status indicates normal functioning of the internal device electronics. If a "--" status is measured along with normal electrode impedance results, the clinician should contact the MED-EL representative for further assessment of the internal device. The quality of coupling is described as "OK," "Weak," "Faint," or "Poor." If there is insufficient coupling between the DIB and the implant, the clinician should reposition the DIB coil over the recipient's implant. In the case of "poor" coupling, the clinician should confirm that the DIB, cable, and coil are adequately connected and functioning properly. If the coupling problem continues, the clinician should contact the MED-EL representative.

The VDP shows voltages measured across all electrodes when stimulating each electrode contact individually and provides a picture of how current fields spread in the cochlea. In the typical case, the voltage distributed to the stimulated electrode contact should be substantially greater than that at any of the other intracochlear electrodes. For example, if electrode 4 is the stimulated electrode contact and the voltage distributed to that electrode is 2.35 volts, the voltage distributed across the other electrodes would be significantly lower than 2.35 volts (i.e., 0.3 volts may be measured across electrode 1). Voltage may be distributed across adjacent electrodes, but the values should be less than 50% of the voltage distributed across the stimulated contact. If voltages distributed across any other channel and the stimulated electrode are similar, it is likely that these two channels are shorted together.

Selecting a Signal Coding Strategy

The next step in the MAESTRO programming platform is to select a signal coding strategy. As described in Chapter 2, there are two MED-EL signal coding strategies: FSP and High Definition CIS (HDCIS). Previous research suggests that the default strategy, FSP, yields better performance and sound quality as well as preference from most recipients. Therefore, the authors recommend initial use of the FSP strategy. If the recipient is not performing well with FSP after several weeks of use, the HDCIS strategy may be used.

In the FSP strategy, pulses on channels that are noted to be "fine structure" will be grouped together into bursts called Channel Specific Sampling Sequences. The onset time of each burst varies with the zero-crossing of the input signal such that the bursts are timed to deliver information that reflects the temporal fluctuations in the input signal. Fine structure information is thus delivered to the most apical channels, and usually between 1 and 3 channels are selected. These are denoted by a music note icon next to the channel number in the programming screen. The actual number of fine structure channels that will be derived in any given program is dependent upon the overall stimulation rate. In the Signal Coding Strategy tab of MAESTRO, the clinician may choose the frequency range for CSSS and the corner frequency above which CSSS will not be implemented; although, MED-EL recommends the default which seeks to maximize the number of CSSS channels. In this tab, the clinician also may set the maximum stimulation rate, which like other strategies, is partially determined by the pulse width on individual channels. The primary unit of stimulation in the MAESTRO software is charge-based, so that the software increases the charge delivered to a particular channel by either increasing amplitude or pulse duration (or both) in response to the clinician's request for more or less stimulation during programming. The goals are to (1) use the narrowest pulse width possible to allow for fast stimulation rates and (2) maximize power efficiency. In the process, the MAESTRO system takes into account electrode impedance as well as the limits of the current source.

Although the MAESTRO platform supports using the highest stimulation rate possible, it is adjustable. However, if the level of stimulation requires the use of a wider pulse width, which is common for most recipients, the stimulation rate will automatically decrease. Higher stimulation rates are possible with deactivation of one or more of the 12 channels. Refer to Chapter 2 for more information on stimulation rate and Chapter 3 for more information on programming considerations related to stimulation rate.

Issues related to voltage compliance also are accessible in the Signal Coding Strategy menu. The Compliance Level Control is an adjustable slider bar that determines how voltage compliance limits are measured. In short, the parameter determines how vigilant the system is at avoiding voltage compliance problems. These may be determined by (1) measured values (i.e., electrode impedance), (2) strict voltage compliance estimation, or (3) theoretical maximum limits using relaxed voltage compliance estimation. The Compliance Level Control default and the typically used setting is Auto Adjust, which seeks to avoid voltage compliance issues and sets pulse width to allow for FSP coding in at least one apical channel. If the user is not experiencing adequate loudness growth with default settings, manual adjustments to the "Compliance Level Control" may improve performance.

Setting Stimulation Levels

In the MAESTRO platform, stimulation levels are adjusted in charge units (qu), but clinical units (cu) also are displayed. Charge units are defined as the product of the amplitude of the stimulus current and the pulse width divided by 1000 [i.e., charge unit = (amplitude of current × pulse width/1000). This unit of stimulation represents constant charge. The system automatically adjusts the amplitude of the stimulus current and/or the pulse to provide the requested loudness while avoiding voltage compliance limits and to maximize stimulation rate. The range of stimulation levels are approximately 0 to 282.2 qu.

It is best to measure stimulation levels on all possible channels; however, an automatic interpolation feature is available in the MAESTRO software. The electrical threshold is referred to as "THR" and is defined as the highest level at which a response is not obtained. As such, the clinician could obtain threshold via typical audiological procedures and set the THR value one or two steps below the measured value; although, how far THR is set below measured threshold is not a critical decision. Many clinicians set THR at 10% of MCL or at minimum levels. Previous research shows similar performance is achieved when using a THR set to 10% of the upper stimulation level versus a measured THR (Spahr & Dorman, 2005). The "lock THR to" option is selected on the right hand side of the Levels screen and will automatically set thresholds to a level determined by the clinician (10% of MCL, 0, etc.). It is important that the level set is completely inaudible to the patient. Thresholds set to an audible level can sometimes result in a buzzing noise in quiet environments. This happens because the coding strategies in the MED-EL system stimulate all activated channels with every frame of data; if a channel does not have any information in it during a frame of stimulation, then that channel is stimulated at the THR level. At default settings, THR is measured using 300 msec bursts of electrical pulses, but it is common practice to create programs with estimated THR levels. When estimated THR levels are used, the stimulation levels for low-level inputs are based on the measured upper stimulation levels.

As previously mentioned, adequate audibility for soft sounds may be determined by measuring soundfield detection thresholds in the audiometric test booth. If soundfield thresholds are elevated (>25–30 dB HL), the clinician could consider increasing MCL values, selecting a steeper MAPLAW function, or measuring THR levels. After this programming change is made, soundfield measurements should be repeated to confirm adequate access to low-level sounds. Additional parameters to improve audibility of low-level sounds will be discussed in the following sections. Finally, if the patient notes a humming sound, especially in quiet environments, it is an indication that at least one threshold value is set to an audible level. The clinician needs to identify the channel that has an audible threshold and lower the THR level to a point where it is not audible to the patient.

The upper level of stimulation, MCL, refers to the maximum level of stimulation that is perceived as loud, but not uncomfortable. When measured with a psychophysical approach, the recipient completes loudness scaling while 50 msec bursts of electrical biphasic pulses are delivered to a single electrode contact. Refer to Chapter 3 for information on determination of upper stimulation levels. MED-EL strongly advocates the use of ESRT as a guide for setting MCL for patients who are unable to respond behaviorally to setting an MCL level. ESRT can be obtained in the normal fitting screen, but a special platform in MAESTRO provides a method to track and better manage ESRT measurements. In the ESRT platform, the stimulus burst has a longer duration (i.e., 500 msec at default) than the stimulus used to determine MCL. The longer duration of the stimulus will make the stapedial reflex more salient for measurement with the acoustic immittance system. The measured ESRT can be imported into the recipient's program in the Levels screen in the ESRT platform. The ESRT has a strong correlation to MCL (Brickley et al., 2005) and, therefore, the clinician should attempt to measure it in all recipients without tympanostomy tubes or obvious middle ear dysfunction. Additional information on ESRT measurements is provided in Chapter 3.

When ESRT cannot be measured, loudness balancing may be conducted at MCL across the electrode array. The Maestro software includes a Sweep function for providing stimulation in a sequential manner across the electrode array. Sweeping may be conducted at the end of the session to ensure that all MCLs are set to equal loudness across the array; it also can be used to ensure the absence of any nonauditory side effects on each channel. Finally, when activating in live speech mode, the clinician may choose the percentage of the electrical dynamic range where stimulation will be presented. Ultimately, the authors recommend a setting of 100% because it is similar to what will be used in the user's typical program. However, for new users, it is necessary to gradually progress to that user level.

Additional Programming Parameters

Frequency Bands. The Frequency Bands screen allows the clinician to control how input sound frequencies are allocated across the active channels. As stated in Chapter 1, MED-EL has the longest electrode array, which provides access to more apical sites of the cochlea. As a result, the MAESTRO software has a low cut-off of 70 Hz in the range of frequencies (i.e., 70 to 8,500 Hz) allocated across the channels. The lower end of the frequency range can be adjusted in 10 Hz steps from 70 to 350 Hz (default = 100 Hz for FSP strategies), while the upper end of the range can be adjusted in 500 Hz steps from 3,500 to 8,500 Hz (default = 8500 Hz). Setting the upper end of the frequency range slightly lower (e.g., 7,000 Hz) may be beneficial because it will create channels with narrower bandwidths in the speech frequencies. Narrower channel bandwidths could improve speech recognition.

Frequencies within the defined input range are reallocated to existing channels using one of four approaches. The default and recommended allocation for the majority of participants is Logarithmic FS," in which the input frequencies are assigned to logarithmically spaced bands. The second option, LinLog, separates the lower frequencies into linear bands and the higher frequencies into logarithmic bands. This mode results in narrower low-frequency bands, which will likely provide better spectral resolution in the low frequencies. Improved spectral resolution may be helpful for discriminating common speech and environmental sounds. The Tonotopic approach attempts to mimic the tonotopic organization observed in the normal cochlea. Theoretically, this mode will produce the most normal frequency percept. Finally, Linear Increasing divides the input frequencies into linear bands with increased bandwidth from the apical to basal direction. This strategy results in wider bandwidths for low-frequency channels relative to Logarithmic FS, but the highest-frequency channels are narrower. This mode may be helpful if the recipient exhibits confusion patterns with high-frequency sounds (e.g., /f/ vs. /s/ vs. /h/). The Frequency Band screen allows the clinician to reorder how channels are allocated to electrode contacts, which is necessary (and should be performed first) when programming a split electrode.

Maplaw. The Maplaw screen allows the clinician to control the logarithmic function used to map acoustic inputs into the recipient's electrical dynamic range. The default choice in the Maplaw menu is Logarithmic Maplaw, which maps lower-level inputs to a higher point in the electrical dynamic range. The other logarithmic function, S-shaped Maplaw, provides less amplification for low-level sounds and a steep increase in amplification for moderate and high-level inputs. The S-shaped Maplaw can be helpful in controlling constant background noise and can be used with patients who need to manage a specific noisy situation (i.e., sitting near a ventilation fan at work).

The clinician also may adjust the default compression coefficient (i.e., 500) used to define the logarithmic function. Higher coefficients map softer inputs to a higher point in the electrical dynamic range. The authors recommend using the compression coefficient of 1000 as soon as it is tolerable for the recipient. Often, at initial stimulation, a maplaw of 1000 will be perceived as too "crisp" or "sharp." In this case, the clinician may need to wait until the patient has a few days of experience with the system before attempting to use a higher maplaw. Long-term, improved audibility of low-level sounds should improve performance.

Volume Mode. The two volume options on the sound processor include the IBK (Innsbruck) and

RTI (Research Triangle Institute) modes. With the IBK default mode, volume control settings correspond to stimulation at a percentage of the electrical dynamic range 0 to 100%. Two parameters can be adjusted in the IBK mode, "minimum" and "maximum" volume control effects, which determine the overall range of the volume control. The minimum and maximum parameters denote the level that will be presented when the volume is turned all the way down or up, respectively. For most patients, the range should be set from 0 to 100%. A narrower range can be used to deactivate the volume control, which may be helpful for children and adults who cannot reliably adjust their volume controls. In addition, the volume buttons on the FineTuner remote control can be deactivated.

The RTI volume control mode is rarely used by clinicians. At the minimum position, no stimulation is provided. As the volume control is increased, the minimum and maximum stimulation levels are increased toward THR and MCL, respectively. One disadvantage of the RTI mode is that some inputs may be inaudible when lower volume settings are used.

Automatic Sound Management (ASM). The ASM screen allows the clinician to adjust input processing characteristics of the system, such as automatic gain control (AGC). Within the ASM menu, the two parameters that may be adjusted include compression ratio and microphone sensitivity. The compression ratio of the AGC system may be disabled or set to one of four ratios (i.e., 2:1, 2.5:1, 3:1, or 3.5:1). The default ratio is 3:1. A lower ratio may be selected if the user reports that loud sounds are too soft (e.g., music); higher ratios may address reports that loud sounds are uncomfortable (although this complaint also should prompt the clinician to re-evaluate and possibly decrease MCL levels). The microphone sensitivity may be adjusted over a range from 0 to 100%. Higher sensitivity settings will provide better audibility of very soft sounds that are close by; however, moderate-level sounds may be too loud, and performance in noise may deteriorate. In contrast, lower sensitivity settings may improve performance and comfort in noise, but soft sounds will not be audible. The default setting of 50% is appropriate for most recipients. The patient can control sensitivity with the FineTuner remote control.

Indicators. The Indicators screen controls warning signals (e.g., low battery beep) and confirmation beeps (e.g., switching programs). The clinician can disable all alerts and control the loudness of enabled alerts according to user preferences.

Programming Previous Generations of MED-EL Implants

All MED-EL recipients with COMBI 40+ and later internal devices may use the OPUS 2 sound processor with the most recent MED-EL signal coding strategies. If the recipient has a COMBI 40+, internal implant with a TEMPO+ or CIS+ sound processor, the sound processor is programmed in the CI.STUDIO+ software platform. However, MAESTRO and CI.STUDIO+ are similar with only a few major differences. First, the user must use CIS+ rather than the FSP sound coding strategy. Second, stimulation levels are measured in clinical units rather than charge units, which

means the clinician has independent control over amplitude and pulse duration on a channel-by-channel basis.

KEY CONCEPTS

The following key concepts were covered in Chapter 4:

- Several adjustable parameters differ across the manufacturers.
- New internal and external devices, and often new processor programming platforms, are released every few years, but many of the manufacturer-specific parameters will be applicable to future processors.
- To supplement the information in this chapter, the reader is encouraged to examine these parameters in the software and contact the manufacturers' representatives for updated information about new parameters, devices, and programming platforms.

‖ 5 ‖

Clinical Considerations: Putting All of the Pieces Together

The previous chapters in this text introduced the basic components of programming a cochlear implant. The objective of this chapter is to assimilate the information into a practical guide for creating successful programs for cochlear implant recipients. General information also is provided on recipient counseling, habilitation/rehabilitation, and interdisciplinary teaming.

COLLABORATION WITH THE COCHLEAR IMPLANT SURGEON/ MEDICAL EVALUATION

Prior to the initial activation of the sound processor, the clinician should inquire about pre-operative and postoperative imaging results and the medical evaluation from the cochlear implant surgeon. Preimplant imaging studies, such as Computed Tomography (CT) or Magnetic Resonance Imaging (MRI), will reveal any abnormalities within the cochlea. For instance, ossification or fibrous tissue growth in the cochlea may occur for patients who are post-meningitic. Ossification may prevent full insertion of the electrode array into the cochlea or elevate the requisite stimulation levels.

Additionally, these imaging studies will reveal the presence of a common cavity cochleae or Mondini's dysplasia. These conditions also may prevent a full insertion as well as be associated with higher stimulation levels, fluctuating stimulation needs, and nonauditory side effects (i.e., facial nerve stimulation).

An MRI also may show the status of the auditory nerve. Several recent publications suggest that some children with congenital deafness are born with aplastic auditory nerves (i.e., absent or severely deficient auditory nerves; Buchman et al., 2006; Rance, 2005), which certainly would result in diminished outcomes and success with a cochlear implant. However, in many of these cases, the aplasia was unilateral. Identification of unilateral aplasia would be critical in selecting the ideal ear for implantation.

The clinician also should inquire about any postoperative x-rays that were conducted to evaluate the status of the electrode array insertion. This information is very important as it indicates how many stimulating electrode contacts are inserted into the cochlea and any extracochlear electrode contacts that should be disabled. Finally, the clinician should query the cochlear implant surgeon about any other surgical/postsurgical complications. Recipients with complications may exhibit anxiety at the activation appointment and often will benefit from positive encouragement from the programming clinician.

At the initial activation and all remaining appointments, the clinician must perform a visual examination of the incision site, an inspection of the area where the transmitting coil will be placed, and an otoscopic examination to rule out the presence of purulent middle ear effusion. Most clinics activate the sound processor 2 to 4 weeks after surgery to allow the incision site to heal and for the resolution of otitis media with serous effusion in the middle ear space, which is not uncommon a few weeks post surgery. At the activation appointment, inspection of the skin is important to ensure that the magnet strength in the external transmitting coil is appropriate. When it is too strong, it may cut off blood flow around the coil and compromise the health of the skin underneath the coil. A medical referral is warranted for trauma at the incision site, persistent purulent otitis media, or otitis media with serous effusion that persists beyond 6 weeks postactivation.

PROGRAMMING SCHEDULE

Two-Day Initial Activation Sessions

As previously mentioned, the optimal stimulation levels for a recipient normally change over the first few weeks or months of cochlear implant use. As a result, frequent programming appointments are necessary to ensure maximum performance and benefit. After the first year of implant use, fewer appointments are necessary.

A recipient's sound processor typically is activated 2 to 4 weeks after cochlear implant surgery. This waiting period provides an opportunity for the incision site and skin flap to heal and for resolution of any serous effusion in the middle ear space. For all recipients, sound processor activation should be divided into two consecutive days. As shown in Table 5–1, a 2-hour session should be scheduled for the first day and 1½-hour session for the second day. The second day allows the recipient to provide feedback to the clinician about early experiences, and the clinician can use this feedback to make adjustments and fine-tune the programming of the sound processor.

On Day 1, after the physical examination, the clinician will determine the appropriate magnet strength to support adhesion of the external transmitting coil to the recipient's head. Young children and elderly women often exhibit thin skin flaps and require relatively weak magnets. Middle-aged men and patients who are obese, however, usually have thick skin flaps and require strong magnets. For users with very thick skin flaps, it may be helpful to shave the hair directly underneath the transmitting coil. For very thin skin flaps, it may be helpful to place a layer of mole skin on the underneath side of the transmitting coil to provide cushion between the coil and skin. Determination of the correct magnet develops with experience; however, the manufacturers provide guidelines on typical magnet strength for children and adults. Although the clinician may be tempted to select a magnet strength that prevents the coil from ever falling off the recipient's head, it is normal for the coil to occasionally detach during rigorous physical activity (e.g., gymnastics, basketball, wrestling, or rough child's play). A magnet with an appropriate strength should be selected cautiously to avoid blood flow restriction to the skin over the internal device. This restriction could result in a skin flap breakdown and the possible need for internal device removal. If the clinician can hold the external coil several inches from the side of the recipient's head and the transmitting coil is aggressively drawn to the internal magnet, the coil is likely too strong. However, if the transmitting coil falls off the user's head several times during programming, the magnet is obviously too weak.

Regardless of the initial magnet strength, the clinician visually should examine the skin flap at every clinical visit. If any sign of irritation occurs or a very prominent impression of the coil can be seen in the user's skin, the magnet strength should be reduced. Adult users may be advised to reduce their own magnet strength if they feel tightness or discomfort around the coil site. Care-

Table 5–1. Overview of Two-Day Activation Appointments

Time Postsurgery	Duration	Basic Overview of Typical Procedures
2 to 4 weeks	2 hours	• Visual examination of incision site and otoscopy • Counsel caregiver to monitor incision site • Basic information: early expectations, use, care, volume control, and batteries • Determine processor magnet strength • Measure impedance at electrode contacts • Select signal coding strategy and base parameters • Determine T levels, USL, volume control
2 to 4 weeks	1.5 hours	• Visual examination of incision site and otoscopy • Additional information: proper use, care, habilitation/ rehabilitation, and telephone use • Demonstrate mastery of basic processor functions • Adjust stimulation levels, measure ESRT* and ECAP • Frequency-specific programming • Adjust and fine-tune programming, restrict volume control

Notes: *if recipient will tolerate procedure; ECAP = electrically evoked compound action potential; ESRT = electrically evoked stapedius reflex threshold; T = threshold levels; USL = upper stimulation levels.

givers of child recipients should be counseled to routinely monitor the status of the incision site. If the child's hair is cut substantially, the caregivers should monitor the skin flap closely for several days following initial activation.

After the magnet is selected for the transmitting coil, the user's sound processor is connected to the programming computer via a device-specific interface. When the programming computer indicates successful communication with the recipient's internal device, the clinician will measure impedance of the stimulating and reference electrode contacts. The programmer must disable identified short or open electrode circuits. The audiologist then must select the appropriate signal coding strategy and initial parameters. Refer to Chapter 4 for direction on choosing signal coding strategies and various adjustable parameters for each implant system.

Next, the clinician will need to remind the patient about realistic expectations in the early stages of cochlear implant use. For an adult recip-

ient, a suggested discussion is as follows: "Remember, when we turn your cochlear implant on today, you may not be entirely pleased with the sound you receive. In fact, you may leave here today thinking, 'I've made a big mistake.' Also, when we first turn it on, many people say that voices sound much different from what they remember with better hearing. Some people note that voices sound cartoonish (like a chipmunk), mechanical, or robotic. In some instances, recipients comment that speech sounds more like beeps or noise. Don't worry. As we've discussed before, it will take the hearing centers of your brain some time to adjust to this new signal. You should notice considerable improvement in sound quality and speech understanding over the next few weeks and months. It will just take time and experience to reach that point. So, the main point today is to not panic or get too upset if the initial sound you receive is less than ideal."

For the caregivers of young children, the conversation immediately prior to activation will be different and may go as follows: "Remember, the initial response a young child shows to sound from a cochlear implant varies widely from child to child. Some children may cry or become upset. It's unlikely that the sound is uncomfortably loud; they are simply unsettled by hearing sounds they've never experienced before. Other children may smile, wave, or point to their ear. In many cases, a child's first responses are subtle. For instance, they may stop playing with the toys, they may glance at you, me, or the programming clinician, they may change their sucking pattern on their pacifier, or they may slightly change their facial expression. Finally, on occasion, children may exhibit very limited responses. Regardless of your child's initial response, remember that it is not at all indicative of how they will eventually perform with the cochlear implant. Also, please remember that your child's auditory skill level is similar to that of a newborn; therefore, sound will have little meaning today. It will take time for the brain to associate meaning with signals from the cochlear implant. As a result, the early responses may be very inconsistent and less than what you might have hoped for. Take heart in the fact that we fully expect your child to benefit from the implant with time and experience."

After the signal-coding parameters and expectations are established, the programming audiologist will determine appropriate stimulation levels for the recipient. Refer to Chapter 3 for a detailed description of measuring threshold and upper stimulation levels. During the first two days of activation, it may be difficult for the adult patient to respond to programming stimuli at threshold (i.e., T level) because of inexperience with electrical stimulation and constant tinnitus. For young, prelingually deafened children with limited to no experience with sound, initial thresholds are likely minimal response levels and are suprathreshold in nature. As a result, the actual T levels are likely to be slightly lower than the measured minimal response levels. It is often necessary to provide a small global decrease in T levels from the values measured to programming stimuli. The child's T level responses to programming stimuli may include changes in sucking patterns and/or facial expressions, a time-locked head turn to the stimulus, a glance toward the parent, clinician, or assis-

tant, a change in play, smiling, pointing to his or her ear, crying, etc. Parents and assistants should help the clinician observe these subtle responses.

For measurement of upper stimulation levels, the authors strongly recommend that parents and caregivers watch their child for signs of discomfort. If a child becomes uncomfortable, the clinician should exercise caution with continued increases in stimulation to avoid overstimulation. Excessively loud stimulation is unpleasant for adults, but it may complicate the early stages of implant use for young children. Specifically, if the child associates the cochlear implant with an unwanted or unpleasant percept, he or she may refuse to wear it. Therefore, when initially activating the implant in live speech mode, threshold and upper stimulation levels should be set at a low level and increased slowly as the clinician or family member talks to and observes the reaction of the recipient. For young children, T levels are fixed at the initial-measurement level. However, after a response is obtained, increases to upper stimulation levels should continue slowly while the child's response is observed.

The final upper stimulation levels for children are based on numerous factors including typical stimulation levels of the cochlear implant system, behavioral responses during programming, electrically evoked stapedial reflex thresholds (ESRT), and observations made during live speech mode. For instance, in the Nucleus 5 system, try to set the upper stimulation levels at least 40 clinical units above the T levels. However, if a child is uncomfortable with these levels, a reduced dynamic range is used for the initial program(s). Remember, the primary goal of the activation appointment for a young child is to facilitate bonding with the implant by providing an audible and comfortable signal across the frequency range, not to create the perfect program. As a colleague of ours is fond of stating, "The process of developing spoken language and auditory skills for a young cochlear implant recipient is not a sprint, but rather a marathon." Given the importance of consistent audibility during the critical period of language development, it is necessary to move quickly toward the optimal program for a child. However, the entire "26.2 miles of the marathon" need not be completed during the first day. Ideally, the clinician will seek to achieve optimal stimulation levels by the one-month postactivation appointment.

For adult recipients, it is important to establish expectations for how speech and environmental sounds likely will be perceived when the sound processor is initially activated in live speech mode. The following instructions may be provided to the recipient: "We are now ready to turn on your cochlear implant so you can hear speech and other environmental sounds. We will start at a very soft volume level, and you most likely will not hear anything at first. After that, we will very slowly increase the volume until you can hear. At first, you may hear a buzzing or ringing sound from the implant. Don't worry. This sound will stop after you wear the implant for a short time and your program settings are optimized."

When live speech first becomes audible, an adult may initially complain. To address this complaint, the clinician may temporarily decrease upper stimulation levels; however, it is best to leave the stimulation on. In many cases, the slow increases to the upper stimulation levels will result in better sound quality. The adult recipient should be asked to indicate what volume setting elicits the most comfortable listening level. In the authors' experience, the initial level selected by the recipient is not the most ideal level; therefore, it may be more desirable to continue slowly increasing stimulation in small step sizes and ask the adult to indicate when the signal is too loud. The clinician may tell the patient, "I am going to increase the volume by a small amount to see if it makes your implant sound better. If it is too loud, then we will turn the volume back down." From this point, the clinician then may decrease the upper stimulation levels by two to five clinical units and confirm that the sound quality is satisfactory. In many cases, recipients request an increase in stimulation levels after acclimating to the sound of the cochlear implant for a day. In other cases, the user may report that certain sounds are too loud. If this occurs, the clinician may decrease upper stimulation levels in the corresponding frequency range or recounsel the recipient about using the volume control. Furthermore, some users will report hearing some sounds (e.g., low-frequency sounds) but struggling to hear others

(e.g., high-frequency sounds). In this case, the clinician can make frequency-specific programming changes to alleviate the difficulties. Finally, at the end of every programming clinician, the clinician may wish to ensure that the recipient can at least detect, if not discriminate, all six Ling sounds. This step ensures sufficient audibility for sounds throughout the speech frequency range (see Chapter 3).

During the first few weeks of cochlear implant use, it is wise to provide a full range for the volume control for the adult and child recipient. This allows them to initially place the transmitting coil on the head with a minimal amount of stimulation and provides flexibility in stimulation to suit their needs. This is especially appropriate for children. Access to volume control is especially important for young children. Specifically, the volume control can be set to the minimum position when the processor and coil is placed on the head and increased to the level deemed appropriate in the programming session within a few seconds. If the child reacts negatively to the sound, the volume is set temporarily to a comfortable level. The caregiver should attempt to increase the volume setting to the preferred setting throughout the first day of use. The volume control is always capped so that the upper stimulation levels provided within a given program will not exceed what was considered appropriate in the programming session.

Another common practice at the early stages of cochlear implant use is to provide the recipient with multiple programs with successively greater stimulation levels. This is especially helpful for people who exhibit significant tolerance problems during the first two days of activation. For instance, in the Nucleus CP810 processor, four programs may be provided with a 3 to 5 clinical unit increase from one program to the next. In the Advanced Bionics and MED-EL systems, multiple programs with progressive global increases in upper stimulation levels will also allow the recipient flexibility to increase total stimulation level. The recipient or family caregiver is encouraged to try to progress through each of the four programs by the next programming session. Again, if the recipient exhibits signs of distress at any program, the previous program should be used. Furthermore, if program #1 is too loud for the recipient, the volume control setting can be reduced from the recommended setting. Finally, if the clinician is satisfied with the stimulation levels that the user will tolerate at the initial activation session, it is not necessary to provide multiple programs. Situation-specific programs (e.g., noise, telephone, music) are not typically introduced until after at least one full week of cochlear implant use to allow the recipient and family to master the more basic functions of the cochlear implant.

To aid in the determination of appropriate stimulation levels during the two-day activation process, the clinician may choose to complete objective measures of cochlear implant function including the ESRT and the electrically evoked compound action potential (ECAP). As previously mentioned, the ESRT is an excellent tool to establish appropriate upper stimulation levels. However, due to the high-level stimulus necessary to elicit the ESRT, some recipients (i.e., young children) may not tolerate this testing during the first two days of activation. During the first several sessions, the acoustic immittance probe should be placed in the ear contralateral to the cochlear implant. If the user received simultaneous bilateral cochlear implants, the clinician should conduct otoscopy and tympanometry and place the immittance probe in the ear with the best admittance. If the ESRT is not obtained in the selected ear, it may be worthwhile to re-measure the ESRT in the opposite ear if it has reasonable admittance at the tympanic membrane.

The stimulus used for ECAP possesses a much lower stimulation rate than the stimuli used for programming and live speech. This lower rate results in a softer loudness percept at an equivalent level of stimulation (i.e., clinical unit/charge unit) because of temporal summation. As a result, most recipients can tolerate the measurement of the ECAP on some channels during the first two days of use. The ECAP measurement system is referred to as Auditory Response Telemetry (ART), Neural Response Imaging (NRI), and Neural Response Telemetry (NRT) in the MED-EL, Advanced Bionics, and Cochlear Corporation systems, respectively. The clinical utility of the ECAP is discussed later in this chapter.

Finally, the clinician must counsel the recipient and his or her family about care, use, and maintenance of the cochlear implant equipment. Recipients often become overwhelmed if every single aspect of the external equipment is discussed during the first day (e.g., accessories, warranty, implications for MRI, etc.). For this reason, the authors recommend discussing and reviewing the basics of implant use during the first two days and more advanced topics at subsequent programming sessions. It is helpful to have the recipient or a family member demonstrate mastery of the most basic functions, such as powering the processor on and off, adjusting the volume control, and changing the batteries. Table 5–2 provides a suggested schedule for discussing various topics throughout the first few weeks of cochlear implant use. Furthermore, the manufacturers provide excellent literature and videos describing the use, care, and maintenance of the cochlear implant along with contraindications for medical procedures. Finally, it is beneficial to provide some basic aural habilitation/rehabilitation during the first two days of activation. Specific suggestions are provided later in this chapter.

One-Week Postactivation Appointment

Following the two-day activation appointment, children and adults should come back for a one-week postactivation appointment to adjust programming parameters. This appointment and all subsequent appointments are scheduled for 60 to 90 minutes depending up on the needs of the recipient. Bilateral cochlear implant recipient appointments are scheduled for 90 to 120 minutes. The week-long experience with the cochlear implant will (1) provide useful information to the clinician to guide programming changes and (2) allow adults and older children to be more effective listeners when behavioral responses are required. Furthermore, recipients usually are able to tolerate higher levels of stimulation and objective measures (i.e., ESRT, ECAP).

At this appointment, the clinician should begin with otoscopy to rule out any external or middle ear pathology and an inspection of the skin flap and incision. After that, for adult recipients, frequency-specific, soundfield detection thresholds are measured to ensure adequate access to

Table 5–2. Suggested Clinician Discussion Topics for the First Few Programming Sessions

Activation Appointment: Session 1
A. *Basic Processor Operation:* (1) Powering processor on/off; (2) changing and recharging batteries; (3) typical battery life; (4) adjusting volume control; (5) operation of remote control
B. *Wear Schedule:* (1) Importance of full-time use; (2) recommended VC setting and program; (3) for children, instruct parent to decrease processor VC to minimum, place on child's head, and then increase to recommended setting; (4) progressive programs, if provided; (5) importance of monitoring health of incision and coil sites
C. *Listening Strategies:* (1) Age-appropriate listening strategies; (2) creating ideal listening environment
D. *Avoid Processor Damage:* (1) Avoid excessive moisture and sources of static electricity
E. *Misc:* (1) Processor wearing/retention options; (2) contact information, questions/problems
Activation Appointment: Session 2
A. *Discuss Experiences:* Counsel about reported experiences
B. *Basic Processor Operation:* Reiterate basic operation of processor—VC, battery life, etc.
C. *Basic Care, Use, and Maintenance:* (1) Use of dehumidifier; (2) microphone care; (3) integrity of various components/reducing strain on and replacing cables; (4) warranty policies
D. *Basic Troubleshooting and Contraindications:* (1) MRI precautions; (2) avoid monopolar cautery; (3) avoid contact sports with risk of injury and scuba diving below 100 meters
1-Week Session
A. *Discuss Experiences:* Counsel about reported experiences
B. *Basic Processor Operation and Accessories:* (1) Inspect settings to ensure appropriate use; (2) discuss basic operation as necessary; (3) for adults, discuss situations—i.e., specific programs; (4) accessory cables-connecting to remote devices; (5) monitoring earphones
C. *Bacterial Meningitis Vaccination:* Importance of vaccination with recommended schedule
D. *Miscellaneous:* (1) Rehabilitative/habilitative guidance; (2) care of processor in extreme conditions (e.g., sports, exercise, working outside, toddlers)
1-Month Session
A. *Discuss Experiences:* Counsel about reported experiences
B. *Basic Processor Functions:* (1) Inspect settings to ensure appropriate use; (2) discuss basic operation as necessary; (3) importance of functional back-up equipment loaded with current programs, bring to every subsequent appointment; (4) protocol for replacing faulty equipment
C. *Removing Barriers:* (1) Hearing Assistance Technology; (2) ensure adequate telephone abilities; (3) introduce FM system if need additional assistance in challenging listening situations
D. *Future Sessions:* Discuss schedule for future programming appointments

low-level sounds (i.e., ≤30 dB HL warble tones from 250 to 6,000 Hz). When responses fall outside of the expected range, the clinician should make adjustments to improve access to low-level sounds. In most cases, open-set speech recognition is not measured at the one-week appointment unless the patient is doing very well. Audiometric soundfield testing typically is not performed for young children (<7 years) at the one-week postactivation appointment given their limited attention spans. Instead, the clinician should focus on optimization of the program. When the physical examination is complete, electrode impedances should be evaluated. Impedance values likely will decrease substantially from the first day of activation and will begin to stabilize.

Next, the clinician should measure T levels on as many channels as possible to adequately characterize the user's threshold profile across the electrode array. Based on experience, measurement of T levels for children with behavioral observation audiometry (BOA) or visual reinforcement audiometry (VRA) may be more difficult because the programming stimulus is no longer novel. Therefore, it may be challenging to keep young children engaged during this programming session.

When the T-level measurements are complete, the clinician should attempt to measure the ESRT in children and adults. When ESRT cannot be measured for young children, upper stimulation levels are based on behavioral measures (see Chapter 3). If it cannot be measured in adults, upper stimulation levels can be set to the most preferable level in live speech mode and loudness balanced across the electrode array. After equal loudness is achieved at upper stimulation levels, the clinician should determine the global upper stimulation level that provides the optimal sound quality and clarity in live speech mode. Slight increases to the final upper stimulation levels may provide improved sound quality and should cease when the subject reports that the signal is too loud or has poor sound quality. From this level, the upper stimulation levels should be decreased until optimal sound quality is obtained. When a satisfactory program is achieved, the ECAP may be measured for electrodes that were not completed at previous sessions.

If an adult seems to understand the basic function of the sound processor and tolerates appropriate stimulation levels, the clinician may introduce situation-specific programs (e.g., telephone, listening in noise, music) and more advanced program features, such as additional signal coding strategies, stimulation rates, etc. (see Chapters 3 and 4). However, for young children who cannot switch settings, it is ideal to provide one program that is suitable across a variety of environments. If the caregiver reports that the child is still not tolerating appropriate stimulation levels, it may be necessary to continue providing multiple programs with increasing levels of stimulation. If the child is showing no aversion to appropriate stimulation levels and is able to initiate implant use at the recommended volume control setting, the clinician should reduce the range over which the volume control operates. This will result in more precise control of volume adjustment for the child or parent.

If time permits, the clinician may demonstrate the use of accessory items (e.g., personal audio cables, monitoring earphones) and review and expand on the proper care of the system (i.e., use of the dehumidifier). If appropriate stimulation levels still have not been determined for a child at the conclusion of the appointment, the child should be scheduled for another programming session within a week. Otherwise, the user returns in three weeks for a one-month, postactivation check-up. A summary of the procedures in typical one- and three-week appointments are provided in Table 5–3.

One-Month Postactivation Programming Session

By the one-month appointment, the recipient should begin to develop a strong bond with the cochlear implant. The recipient and family usually are able to provide substantial feedback about progress to guide the audiologist in programming changes. Most of the time, postlingually deafened adults will report significant improvements in their ability to understand speech. As a result, aided soundfield detection thresholds and speech recognition are evaluated at the beginning of this session. For users of bilateral implants, thresholds and speech recognition should be measured for each ear. These thresholds and scores contribute to necessary program changes. For example, if detection thresholds are elevated in the high-frequency range (e.g., >25 dB HL, 2,000 to 6,000 Hz), the clinician will focus on programming adjustments to improve access to high-frequency, low-level sounds.

At this point, it is imperative that children are using the cochlear implant during all waking hours. If the parent reports situations other than bath time or swimming in which the cochlear

Table 5–3. Overview of One-Week and Optional Three-Week Postactivation Appointments

Time Postactivation	Duration	Basic Overview of Typical Procedures
1 week	1 hour	• Visually examine incision site, otoscopy, impedances • Measure T levels, ESRT, and ECAP for remaining electrodes • Make adjustments to USL in live speech mode • Child: provide one program • Adult: aided soundfield thresholds; situation-specific programs • Reduce volume control range • Discuss care in greater detail and demonstrate accessories
3-week interim	1 hour	• Only necessary when T and USL levels not yet determined • Visually examine incision site and otoscopy • Protocol similar to 1-week appointment

Notes: ECAP = electrically evoked compound action potential; ESRT = electrically evoked stapedius reflex threshold; T = threshold levels; USL = upper stimulation levels.

implant is not used, the clinician should counsel the family about the importance of full-time implant use. Children's soundfield detection thresholds ought to be evaluated at the beginning of the appointment and should be no poorer than 30 dB HL in the low frequencies and 25 dB HL in the mid- to high frequencies. Programming changes are necessary if these goals are not met. Speech recognition may be evaluated for children older than three years of age who have previous hearing aid experience.

The remainder of the one-month appointment involves the same measures conducted at previous appointments. Otoscopy and examination of the skin flap and incision site are followed by a visual inspection of the sound processor (i.e., signs of wear, tear, or damage). If the sound processor allows, the clinician should perform a biologic listening check with monitor earphones to evaluate the status of the sound processor microphone. Next, the clinician should perform impedance measures and determine T levels and upper stimulation levels. Multiple T-level measurements at several channels will be necessary to determine profile changes across the electrode array. If T levels are relatively constant across the array, they will be measured on only a few electrodes and the remaining values will be inter-polated. However, substantial T level variability warrants measurements on a greater number of channels. Next, upper stimulation levels should be optimized using previously discussed procedures, and the ESRT should be measured. For adults, the volume control should allow for only small adjustments (e.g., –30%/+15 percent of the dynamic range). In children, the upper end of the volume control should not exceed the upper stimulation levels set in the program, and the lower end of the volume control range is dependent upon the child's tolerance for stimulation. If no tolerance problems exist, volume control ought to be disabled or should only allow for minimal decreases in volume (e.g., –20 percent of the dynamic range or less). However, if tolerance problems do exist, the volume control should allow for substantial decreases (i.e., 50 percent or greater of the dynamic range). The final component of the one-month appointment is an introduction of situation-specific programs if not yet completed at the previous session.

Remainder of Programming Schedule

After the one-month appointment, programming schedules differ between adults and children but involve similar procedures and mirror those described for the one-month session. A summary of the steps included in the one- and three-month postactivation appointments is shown in Table 5–4. For children younger than 7 years, two- and three-month postactivation appointments are scheduled to ensure optimal access to low-level sounds and appropriate program settings. Following the three-month appointment, the child should return every three months for assessment of auditory skills, verification of cochlear implant function, and programming. In addition, young children with cochlear implants should receive intensive audition-based therapy/habilitation to optimize auditory and spoken language development. The audiologist should collaborate with the Listening and Spoken Language Specialist (LSLS) or speech-language pathologist to ensure that the child's speech and language is developing appropriately. If concerns arise, more frequent audiologic evaluations and implant-programming sessions may be warranted. When the child reaches 7 years of age and has at least two years of cochlear implant experience,

audiologic assessment and programming are conducted every six months.

Following the one-month postactivation appointment, adults typically return for a three-month programming session. However, if an adult is struggling at the one-month appointment, he or she should be seen for a two-month postactivation appointment. Following the three-month appointment, adults are seen every three months through the first year of implant use and on a biannual or annual basis thereafter. A summary of the appointments following the three-month postactivation session is outlined in Table 5–5.

THE ROLE OF ELECTRICALLY EVOKED POTENTIALS IN PROGRAMMING

Several researchers have described the possible role of electrically evoked surface-measured potentials (i.e., measured from electrodes on the head)

Table 5–4. Overview of One-Month and Three-Month Postactivation Appointments

Time Postactivation	Duration	Basic Overview of Typical Procedures
1 month	1 hour	• Visually examine incision site and otoscopy • Feedback about progress and discuss duration of implant use • Aided soundfield thresholds & speech recognition • Visually examine and biologic listening check on processor • Measure electrode impedances and T levels • Optimize USL; measure ESRT • Reduce volume control range or disable • Provide situation-specific programs
2 and 3 months	1 hour	• Visually examine incision site and otoscopy • Soundfield detection thresholds and speech recognition • Similar procedures as one-month session • Child: Ensure access to soft sounds; determine whether program levels and settings are appropriate • Adult: seen at 2 months if struggling; otherwise, seen at 3 months

Notes: ESRT = electrically evoked stapedius reflex threshold; T = threshold levels; USL = upper stimulation levels.

Table 5–5. Appointment Schedule Following the Three-Month Postactivation Session

Time Postactivation	Duration	Basic Overview of Typical Procedures
Every 3 months	1 hour	• Visually examine incision site and otoscopy • Soundfield detection thresholds and speech recognition • Visual exam and biologic listening check on processor • Measure electrode impedances and ESRT • Adjust T levels, USL, parameters, and programs • Child: assess auditory skills; clinician collaborate with LSLS
Child: Every 6 months	1 hour	• For child 7 years or older with 2 years of implant experience • Visually examine incision site and otoscopy • Soundfield detection thresholds and speech recognition • Procedures similar to 3-month session
Adult: biannual or annual	1 hour	• For adult after 1 year of implant use; dependent on needs • Visually examine incision site and otoscopy • Soundfield detection thresholds and speech recognition • Perform procedures similar to 3-month session

Notes: ESRT = electrically evoked stapedius reflex threshold; LSLS = language and spoken language specialist; T = threshold levels; USL = upper stimulation levels.

in cochlear implant management (Brown, Abbas, Fryauf-Bertschy, Kelsay, & Gantz, 1994; Kileny, 2007; Sharma & Dorman, 2006), but for the most part, these measures are not used in routine clinical practice. There are, however, numerous clinicians who measure the ECAP of the auditory nerve via specialized telemetry measures available in the implant hardware and software. The ECAP is measured when the intracochlear electrode contacts serve to stimulate the auditory nerve and record its responses. It is a fairly simple measure because no additional equipment is required, and it can be measured while the recipient is awake and active. In addition, consistently measuring the ECAP is advantageous because it (1) indicates a stimulus level that definitely should be audible, (2) confirms the responsiveness of the auditory nerve to electrical stimulation, and (3) serves as an objective baseline of physiologic function to which subsequent measurements can be compared.

As previously discussed, the ECAP is used to estimate threshold and upper stimulation levels, and a large amount of variability exists in these relationships. In fact, subjects may have ECAP thresholds that fall near T levels, near upper stimulation levels, or in the middle of their electrical dynamic range. It is difficult to pinpoint the exact cause of this subject variability, but three possibilities include (1) the inter- and intrarecipient differences in the geometrical orientation between the stimulating electrode and recording contacts across the electrode array (has a big impact on the response recorded via a near field approach, such as ECAP with cochlear implants), (2) subject differences in neural refractory properties, and (3) differences among electrode arrays. Given the variability across recipients, a single correction factor is not feasible for estimating program levels from the ECAP.

Some researchers suggest using a combination of ECAP and a set of abbreviated behavioral programming levels to determine stimulation needs across the electrode array (Franck, 2002; Hughes, Brown, Abbas, Wolaver, & Gervais, 2000). For instance, ECAP thresholds are measured across the electrode array, and T and upper stimulation levels are measured for one channel in the middle of the array or three channels spaced at the apical, middle, and basal sites of the array. Although this combined approach yields a more accurate estimation of stimulation needs, the potential for mistakes still exists. For example, Figure 5–1 shows NRT thresholds superimposed over program levels for reliable adults with excellent performance.

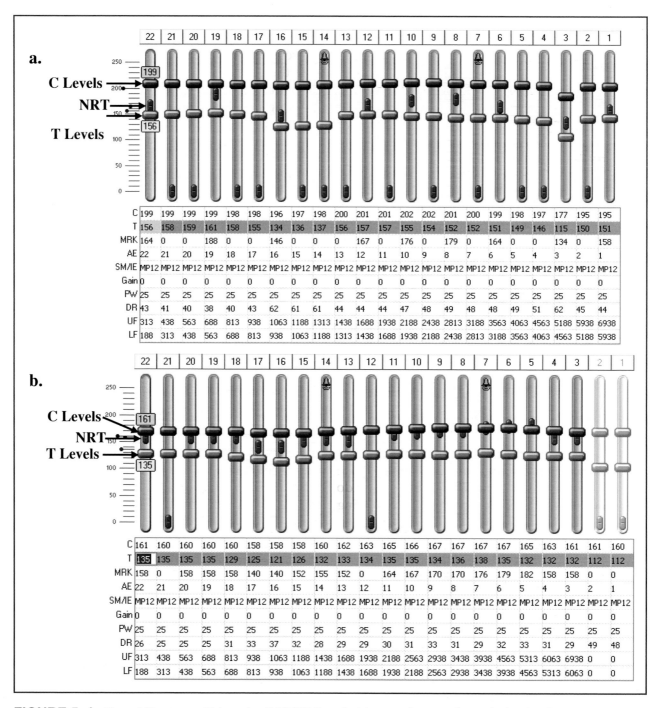

FIGURE 5–1. Neural Response Telemetry (NRT™) thresholds superimposed over behaviorally measured program levels for an adult. (**a**) NRT responses near T levels, (**b**) NRT responses near upper stimulation (C) levels. (Courtesy of Cochlear™ Americas, © 2009 Cochlear Ltd.)

As shown in the two examples, the NRT threshold can approach the upper stimulation level (i.e., C level) for one person and T levels for another. If the clinician was using the combined ECAP/behavioral approach, suboptimal stimulation levels would be provided for this recipient. Given the variable relationship of ECAP to measured stimulation needs, the clinician should exercise extreme caution when using this objective measure. Behavioral and ESRT measures serve as better indicators of ideal program levels. In short, the clinician should continue to bring the recipient in for programming sessions until behavioral measures confirm that the stimulation levels provided by the implant are providing sufficient audibility. When the ECAP must be used as a last resort for estimating program levels, it should be combined with behavioral approaches.

ADDITIONAL HABILITATIVE/REHABILITATIVE CONSIDERATIONS

Developing an ideal program is certainly important for success with a cochlear implant, but receiving specialized audition-based therapy or aural rehabilitation is also important. This specialized therapy or rehabilitation facilitates maximal performance with the device for two reasons. First, the electrical signal from a cochlear implant is much different than the acoustic signal from a hearing aid. Second, auditory skills acquired with cochlear implants are very impressive but still do not match that of a person with normal-hearing sensitivity. Therefore, aural rehabilitation for adult recipients is recommended during the first few weeks or months of cochlear implant use.

The rehabilitation program should be directed by a LSLS or by an audiologist with experience in aural rehabilitation for adults with severe-to-profound deafness. In addition, the cochlear implant manufacturers have developed very effective computer-based aural rehabilitation programs, which are available on their websites or compact disc (CD-ROM). These manufacturer-designed programs are often critical for adults without access to individualized aural therapy but also supplement rehabilitation of adults enrolled in formal programs. The programming audiologist also should be equipped with several rehabilitative tools to facilitate early success with the cochlear implant. For example, when the implant initially is activated in live speech mode, the user is asked to listen as the clinician says the days of the week or months of the year. The clinician stops on a given day or month and asks the user to say the following day/month. In this example, the recipient's auditory memory is used to support the auditory input. Most users can accomplish this exercise, which helps them associate meaning to the sound and builds their confidence with the cochlear implant. Adults also are encouraged to seek out sounds during the first few weeks of cochlear implant use. For example, they can turn on the water faucet to associate meaning to the sound it generates. Recipients also should seek out sounds to which they cannot associate meaning. If they cannot identify a sound, family members or friends should be asked to assist them in identifying its source.

Auditory/visual tracking is another effective rehabilitation activity in the early stages of implant use. In this exercise, the recipient listens and follows along visually as the clinician reads a book, magazine, or newspaper aloud. The clinician stops reading somewhere within the passage, and the recipient is asked to say the next word in the passage. Obviously, recipients may rely on visual input to support the auditory signal from the cochlear implant, but this exercise will help them associate specific words to novel sounds. Familiar phrase cards are also beneficial during initial stages of implant use. Two to four cards are placed on the table, and the clinician reads the phrase or words on one of the cards aloud. Recipients are asked to select the card that was read. This task can begin at the level of pattern perception (i.e., cards having words with different syllable length) and progress to closed-set word identification. Although the previously mentioned exercises seem somewhat elementary, they help to build confidence and auditory-skill level at the initial activation sessions. The aforementioned exercises do not represent a comprehensive aural rehabilitation program for the adult patient. Again, if the programming clinician is not well-versed in audiologic rehabilitation, he or she should consider referral services from a specialist experienced with working with cochlear implant users, particularly when the recipient does not experience rapid success with cochlear implant.

Audition-based habilitation/rehabilitation is absolutely critical for young children with a cochlear implant. Although the programming audiologist can provide support, all children should be managed closely by a LSLS who will guide the child and family toward optimal development of speech, language, and auditory skills. As previously stated, the audiologist should correspond closely with the LSLS to ensure the child's progress. At the initial activation appointment, the programming audiologist is responsible for ensuring that the child's caregivers have a thorough understanding of the use, care, and maintenance of the cochlear implant system as well as the importance of using it during all waking hours. Oral and written instruction should be provided at the initial session, and the audiologist should revisit the basics of implant use at subsequent appointments. In addition, the audiologist and family should determine the most appropriate wearing option for retention of the sound processor to the child's head to body.

On the first day of cochlear implant use, families should be encouraged to walk around the home and point out the different sounds they encounter. For instance, they can knock on the door, point to their ear, and say "I heard that." The LSLS often refers to this activity as a "listening walk," which helps children associate meaning to new sounds. Other examples of sounds on a listening walk include ringing from the telephone, running water, and sounds from toys. If the child appears to respond to speech or an environmental sound, the caregiver should provide enthusiastic positive reinforcement, while pointing to her own ear and saying, "I heard that!" Parents should also be encouraged to provide an oral description of even the most mundane events of life. For example, when walking into a room, the parent should say, "Okay, we're walking in the room, and now we're going to turn on the light. Oh, the light came on." Consistent descriptions of daily activities provide the child with a rich model of speech and language development. Another wonderful exercise to recommend for auditory-skill development in young children is the simple act of reading books. Reading aloud to children serves as an excellent model for language and literacy development.

Finally, caregivers should attempt to optimize the acoustics in the home. For example, if no one is watching the television, it should be turned off to reduce competing noise. Also, to provide a good signal-to-noise ratio during the early stages of implant use, the parent should attempt to remain in close proximity to the child and direct speech to the side of the implant when communicating. Obviously, the aforementioned suggestions are not exhaustive and only introduce a few ideas for building an "auditory lifestyle."

CONSIDERATIONS FOR BILATERAL COCHLEAR IMPLANTATION

The basic fundamentals of cochlear implant programming also apply to the programming of two cochlear implants; however, a few special considerations must be taken into account. First, bilateral cochlear implant programming appointments are time intensive. When recipients receive two cochlear implants in the same surgical procedure (i.e., simultaneous implantation), the initial activation appointments should be increased to 3 hours for the first day and 2 hours for the second day. All subsequent appointments should be scheduled for two hours. Most adults are able to complete both the evaluation of implant function (e.g., booth testing) and cochlear implant programming during one full session. Children under the age of 12, however, often have a difficult time attending to the behavioral tasks for a two-hour session. As a result, two appointments on separate days may be necessary, one hour-long session for behavioral testing and one 60-to-90-minute session for programming. For families who travel a great distance to the programming center, the assessment and programming sessions may be scheduled for the morning and afternoon, respectively. It is very important that the audiologist have a variety of entertaining games and toys available to facilitate conditioned play audiometry and cooperation during objective measures.

Determination of cochlear implant stimulation levels and other adjustable parameters are similar to the practices used for unilateral recipients. The clinician should try to match adjustable parameters, such as stimulation rate, input dynamic range (IDR), and frequency allocation. However, published studies and anecdotal experience suggest that most recipients receive bilateral benefit, even with ear differences (Dorman & Dahlstrom, 2004).

Balancing loudness between the two ears is intuitively appealing, but there are no standardized protocols for how this should be accomplished. Most clinicians query the recipient about the loudness difference between the ears while listening in live speech mode and make global adjustments to upper stimulation levels to achieve a balanced loudness percept between ears. Tyler et al. (2006) describes an alternative approach in which the recipient listens to external, frequency-specific signals (e.g., warble tones or narrowband noise at 500 and 2,000 Hz) presented from 90 and 270 degrees in the horizontal azimuth and reports whether they are matched in loudness or if the right- or left-sided signal is louder. Programming adjustments are made to achieve equal loudness for the signals at each frequency. More research is needed to determine the most effective strategy to optimize bilateral stimulation levels. Many recipients experience bilateral summation with the use of two cochlear implants (Schafer, Amlani, Seibold, & Shattuck, 2007). However, no published studies indicate the standard magnitude of this summation or how it should be managed in the programming process. In most cases, bilateral summation can be addressed by providing a small global decrease in upper stimulation levels relative to those determined in the unilateral conditions. If the decrease results in a significantly reduced electrical dynamic range in one ear, larger decreases to upper stimulation levels may be necessary for the ear with the wider dynamic range.

Following the one-month postactivation appointment, soundfield detection thresholds should be evaluated for each ear separately at the beginning of each session to confirm access to low-level sounds. Because the recipient likely wears both cochlear implants during all waking hours, it may not be apparent that audibility is insufficient for one ear. Speech recognition in quiet and in noise also should be assessed for each ear separately and in the bilateral condition.

These conditions will confirm bilateral benefit, and more importantly, rule out the very rare possibility of bilateral interference.

No consensus exists regarding the most appropriate wearing schedule for people who receive two cochlear implants in separate surgical procedures (i.e., sequential implantation). Clinicians may recommend full-time use of both implants, periods of use with the new cochlear implant alone, or only the newly implanted ear for several weeks. More research is necessary to determine the ideal schedule of implant use for recipients with varying pre-implant histories.

Finally, many cochlear implant recipients wear a hearing aid on the opposite ear (i.e., bimodal arrangement). Once again, it is desirable to balance loudness between the two ears. Information on optimizing the signal of each device is described by Ching and colleagues (Ching, Incerti, & Hill, 2004; Ching, Psarros, Hill, Dillon, & Incerti, 2001).

KEY CONCEPTS

Following this chapter, the reader should recognize concepts associated with the following topics:

- The clinician must consult with the surgeon about the pre- and postimplantation imaging results and other medical needs.
- The cochlear implant activation appointment should be scheduled on two separate days to complete the necessary measurements and assessments.
- The one-week and one-month postactivation appointments should be followed by different appointment schedules for adults and for children.
- Habilitation/rehabilitation is necessary for adults and children to achieve their full potentials with the cochlear implant.
- There are several specific considerations for programming bilateral cochlear implants including the need for increased programming time and balance of adjustable parameters and loudness levels between ears.

III 6 III

Troubleshooting Patient Complaints and Complications

Advances in cochlear implant technology and clinical procedures, expansion of candidacy, and earlier identification of hearing loss in children have resulted in considerable benefit for the overwhelming majority of recipients. In some instances, however, children are not developing age-appropriate speech and language skills, and adults do not achieve excellent open-set speech recognition. Some recipients experience initial difficulties with their cochlear implants, but after adept management by the programming clinician, they achieve substantial benefit. It is fairly common for even the most successful recipients to experience temporary setbacks, which may be attributed to faulty external equipment or minor programming needs. These issues typically are addressed efficiently and effectively by the seasoned programming clinician. The goal of this chapter is to discuss the audiologic management of recipients who experience suboptimal outcomes, complications, and temporary and chronic difficulties. Suggestions also are provided for the management of difficult-to-program recipients.

MANAGING RECIPIENTS WHO EXPERIENCE DISAPPOINTING OUTCOMES

Numerous factors may be responsible for deficient performance with a cochlear implant, but they most often are related to patient characteristics. In other cases, unsatisfactory performance or temporary difficulty may be attributed to an extrinsic factor (e.g., faulty hardware, poor program, etc.). Therefore, the following potential extrinsic causes should be evaluated.

External Hardware

Although the reliability and durability of external hardware has improved over the past few years, malfunction of external components always should be considered as a potential cause for poor patient performance. First, a visual examination of the external hardware should be conducted to check for signs of wear or faults. It is especially important to inspect the transmitting cable(s) for evidence of anomalies as the wires inside the cable often are susceptible to breakage. When the function of the transmitting cables is in doubt, the clinician should ask the recipient to switch to the back-up cable to see whether performance and sound quality improve. For young children who cannot report on the integrity of the signal, the transmitting cables should be replaced every six months. Next, the clinician visually should assess the batteries and battery contacts for signs of corrosion or faults and the appearance of the microphone ports. The water-resistant covers over some sound processor microphones should be clean and free of debris. When possible, the clinician should also assess the microphone function with a listening check (i.e., Cochlear Corporation/Advanced Bionics monitor earphones). As discussed in previous chapters, it is imperative to measure soundfield detection thresholds to ensure that the sensitivity of the microphone allows for access to low-level sounds across the speech-frequency range (i.e., 250–6000 Hz). The clinician then should confirm that the transmitting coil is sending and receiving signals to the internal device using a signal-check wand, a diagnostic remote control (e.g., CR110), or by performing telemetry measure via the computer programming software interface. Furthermore, the clinician should verify that all controls and indicators are functioning properly. Finally, most recipients own a back-up sound processor for troubleshooting purposes, and in the event that performance and progress are poor, the recipient should switch to this back-up device. If the problem is addressed, the clinician systematically should replace each of the sound processor components to identify the faulty link. If the recipient does not have a back-up processor, the clinic's loaner equipment should be used for troubleshooting.

Determine Wear Schedule and Facilitate an Auditory Lifestyle

To achieve the full potential with a cochlear implant, young children must use it during all waking hours, and the family must provide an enriching model for speech, language, and auditory development. Children in families that enforce only sporadic use of the implant, achieve fair progress at best. In addition, children in families that do not stress audition and have limited expectations for spoken language typically will lag far behind the development of their peers with normal hearing.

When inquiring about a wear schedule and the communication lifestyle at home, questions should be worded carefully to elicit a forthright response. If one asks whether the child wears the cochlear implant during all waking hours, the caregiver likely will answer affirmatively, as the question implies that the objective is full-time use. In contrast, an inquiry about the number of times or hours the child "takes a break" from the implant is likely to yield a more accurate estimate from the caregiver. The clinician should gently and tactfully reinforce the importance of full-time cochlear implant use. Likewise, the clinician should inquire about the number and types of visual supports used to assist communication. If the family relies heavily on visual input, the clinician may provide some suggestions for supporting communication through audition-based strategies. Finally, the clinician should correspond with the child's Listening and Spoken Language Specialist (LSLS) to ensure the family is equipped with effective strategies to facilitate listening at home.

For the elderly adult who lives alone, it may be difficult to establish consistent social interaction with friends or loved ones. As previously mentioned, a new recipient requires a period of time to adjust to the new signal. If the user is unable to practice listening and have routine conversations, the progress will be slow and the adjustment of the central auditory system to novel signal from the implant will be delayed. For those with limited social interaction, the clinician should suggest activities or structured therapy to facilitate adjustment to the device.

Evaluate the Appropriateness of the Cochlear Implant Program

When the external equipment is functioning normally and the recipient is using the device properly, the clinician should reevaluate the appropriateness of the user's program. Electrode impedances should be within normal limits, have unremarkable morphology (e.g., no large variability in impedance between contacts), and be similar to previous measurements. Next, the clinician should confirm that threshold (T) levels and upper stimulation levels are set accurately. Of all adjustable program parameters, the threshold and upper stimulation levels will have the greatest influence on patient performance and sound quality. Again, the electrically evoked stapedial reflex threshold (ESRT) serves as the best indicator of appropriate upper stimulation levels (see Chapters 3 and 5).

If the stimulation levels are set appropriately, the clinician may consider revising the signal coding strategy or adjustable program parameters, such as stimulation rate, maxima, and in put dynamic range (see Chapters 3 and 5). Finally, the clinician should obtain objective measures of auditory function (e.g., ECAP) and compare them to previous results to identify any unwanted changes. If degradation is observed, the clinician should schedule a medical evaluation and an integrity assessment of the internal device. When adjustments of the aforementioned parameters are successful, the programming audiologist, recipient, family, and LSLS should notice considerable improvement in performance immediately, but definitely no later than three months.

Assessment of Internal Hardware

When all other factors are ruled out as potential causes of poor progress, the clinician should scrutinize and assess the function of the internal device. All three manufacturers offer technical support in providing relatively thorough assessments of internal device integrity. Many faults are identified successfully with these assessments, but some recipients will have "normal" findings with a faulty internal device.

The clinician also may request that the otologist order another postoperative plain film x-ray to confirm that the internal device has not migrated or moved from its original position. This recommendation is especially warranted for sudden changes in stimulation levels or electrode impedance values. The otologist will determine whether shifts in internal device placement may be responsible for the negative changes in recipient performance.

Finally, recent evidence suggests that more advanced imaging procedures, such as computerized rotational tomography and 64-slice computerized tomography scan imaging, may provide valuable information about electrode array placement and the cochlea's condition after implantation. Specifically, research shows this imaging can be used to determine whether the electrode array has remained in the scala tympani or has dislocated to other chambers within the cochlea (Lane, Driscoll, Witte, Primak, & Lindell, 2007; Postnov et al., 2006). Preliminary research suggests that recipient performance is related inversely to the number of electrodes outside the scala tympani (Finley et al., 2008). This imaging also may be used to identify the presence of fibrous tissue growth or ossification after implantation.

IDENTIFYING "RED FLAGS"

Amy McConkey Robbins introduced the term "red flag" as an indicator of slow or limited recipient progress (Robbins, 2005). A flag occurs when a certain skill lags behind the development of normal-hearing peers or below expectations for a given time period after activation. A red flag signifies the need for more proactive monitoring of pediatric recipient performance, but it is also applicable to adult recipients.

In order to identify a possible red flag, the clinician must be aware of typical progress with a cochlear implant and normal speech and language development. The most desirable objective of cochlear implantation is to allow for communication via spoken language across a variety of listening environments, and this goal is achieved for most recipients. Most children who receive a cochlear implant at a relatively young age (≤3 years) and have normal cognitive and neurological function develop some speech, language, and auditory skills within one year of implant use. This goal also should apply to children who received considerable benefit from hearing aids and received a cochlear implant at a later age. When a child's progress does not meet this benchmark, the cochlear implant team should explore the reason(s) for the limited benefit.

Most adults with postlingual deafness and a limited duration of deafness (i.e., <20 years) develop good-to-excellent, open-set speech recognition and spoken-language skills. In fact, the vast majority of adults who use recent technology and obtain regular audiology services should be able to converse over the phone and achieve ceiling performance (i.e., 100% correct) on open-set sentence-recognition tests after three months of implant use. Certainly, the adult's performance should be significantly better than that obtained with hearing aids immediately prior to implantation. Once again, if these goals are not met, the cochlear implant team actively should explore the reasons for limited progress and suggest means for improved performance.

Factors Influencing Cochlear Implant Outcomes

Outcomes from cochlear implantation are closely related to personal factors (e.g., preimplant hearing, otologic history, age, and family support) and intrapersonal characteristics (e.g., cognitive and neurological status, personal motivation, and use of communication strategies). In addition, previous research suggests variable outcomes for some recipients with additional disabilities, a history of bacterial meningitis, aplastic auditory nerves, inner ear malformations, long durations of deafness (i.e., >20 years and severe high-frequency hearing loss), advanced age, and prelingual deafness. Although the aforementioned patient characteristics may influence performance, they should not be considered as absolute contraindications for cochlear implan-

tation. We have personal experience with recipients in each of these categories who still show remarkable benefit from a cochlear implant. Finally, performance certainly will be influenced if the integrity of the internal cochlear implant is compromised.

Additional Disabilities

Approximately 40% of children with hearing loss have an additional disability. Many of these children do well with a cochlear implant, but a low nonverbal intelligence or depressed neurological or cognitive status may have deleterious effects on the development of spoken-language skills. Examples of conditions that are known to limit spoken-language development in children are below average intelligence, mental retardation, autism, and neurological effects associated with Cytomegalovirus (CMV). The extent to which these conditions impact cochlear implant outcomes is directly related to the severity of the associated neurological and cognitive deficits. When additional disabilities are identified prior to surgery, it is important for the audiologist to discuss the potential for diminished outcomes following implantation. Even when a young child does not exhibit any obvious secondary disability, it is good practice to counsel families that speech and language outcomes often are impacted by neurological and cognitive status. Specific guarantees to parents regarding outcomes cannot and should not be made.

Bacterial Meningitis

Published reports indicate mixed cochlear implant outcomes for children who were deafened secondary to bacterial meningitis (Durisin, Arnoldner, Stover, Lenarz, & Lesinski-Schiedat, 2008; Mitchell, Psarros, Pegg, Rennie, & Gibson, 2000). Some of the children in these studies had similar speech and language outcomes as compared to the general pediatric cochlear implant population. For this reason, an etiology of bacterial meningitis should not prevent cochlear implantation. However, other subjects had poorer outcomes than the typical pediatric population with cochlear implants, which likely are related to cochlear ossification or neurological deficits. A full insertion of the electrode array may not be achieved in recipients with significant ossification. First, ossification may result in significant degeneration of spiral ganglion dendrites and adversely may affect the delivery of electrical current from the electrode contacts to the auditory nerve. Second, it is well known that bacterial meningitis may cause significant neurological insults. When this occurs, language outcomes will be affected. Finally, for children with a history of bacterial meningitis, reduced outcomes may occur if duration of deafness before implantation is longer than 6 months (Durisin et al.). During this 6-month period, the potential for significant ossification is high; therefore, the surgeon may not achieve a full electrode array insertion. As a result, cochlear implantation should occur as soon as possible following deafness secondary to bacterial meningitis.

Aplastic Auditory Nerves

An emerging body of literature suggests poorer outcomes for cochlear implant recipients who have absent or severely deficient auditory nerves as compared to those with other etiologies (Walton, Gibson, Sanli, & Prelog, 2008), and other research shows no differences in outcomes between groups (Jeong, Kim, Kim, Bae, & Kim, 2007; Peterson et al., 2003). This condition may be associated with a preimplant diagnosis of auditory neuropathy spectrum disorder (ANSD). Contemporary magnetic resonance imaging (MRI) can determine the status and integrity of the auditory nerve prior to implantation. This imaging is warranted for children with ANSD or limited responses on behavioral and objectives assessments of auditory function. Identification of a unilateral cochlear nerve deficiency would be critical for determining the most appropriate ear for implantation (Buchman et al., 2006). Although outcomes associated with cochlear nerve deficiency are typically poor, the family may choose to move forward with cochlear implantation. In this case, the family should be counseled that spoken-language outcomes may be poorer than expected, the implant may improve only sound

awareness, and they should support a visually based communication mode (i.e., sign language). The electrically evoked transtympanic auditory brainstem response (ABR) assessment may serve as a prognostic indicator of the system's ability to respond to electrical stimulation in a synchronous manner (Gibson, Sanli, & Psarros, 2009; Kileny & Zwolan, 2004).

Inner Ear Malformations

Unlike the previously mentioned conditions, children with inner ear malformations often have successful cochlear implant outcomes (Buchman et al., 2004; Loundon et al., 2005). For example, children with enlarged vestibular aqueduct syndrome typically perform as well or better than the general pediatric population with cochlear implants (Bent, Chute, & Parisier, 1999). Children with Mondini malformations also do well with cochlear implants, but the outcome generally is related to the extent of the malformation (Arnolder et al., 2004; Buchman et al.). Finally, many children who have common cavity deformities experience positive outcomes with cochlear implants (Buchman et al.), but they have more complications than children with less involved cochlear deformities (Mylanus, Rotteveel, & Leeuw, 2004). Because stimulation levels are more likely to fluctuate for this population, more frequent programming and assessment appointments are necessary (i.e., every 3 months).

Prelingual Deafness and Duration of Deafness Prior to Implantation

Adults with prelingual deafness and limited listening and spoken-language experience often exhibit poorer outcomes when compared to adults with postlingual deafness. Numerous studies show limited open-set speech recognition and poorer spoken-language abilities for adults with prelingual deafness (Kaplan, Shipp, Chen, Ng, & Nedzelski, 2003; Teoh, Pisoni, & Miyamoto, 2004). In addition, some teenagers with prelingual deafness eventually may become nonusers because of limited benefit, cosmetic issues, or peer pressure. However, an implant almost certainly will improve detection of speech and environmental sounds, and speech perception will improve relative to preimplant scores (Santarelli, De Filippi, Genovese, & Arslan, 2008). Adults and teenagers in this category must be self-motivated to pursue a cochlear implant and have realistic expectations. If the potential candidate's family serves as the primary impetus toward cochlear implantation, the likelihood of a poor outcome and limited implant use is even greater. As such, the clinician should provide deliberate and truthful information regarding realistic expectations for this population in the candidate's preferred communication modality. If the user has realistic expectations and wishes to pursue a cochlear implant to enhance sound detection and support manual communication, the person may be considered for implantation.

In addition to limitations associated with prelingual deafness, several researchers report that durations of deafness exceeding 5 years may negatively influence cochlear implant outcomes (Green et al., 2007; Oh et al., 2003), but certainly exceptions to this rule can be found. As the duration of deafness begins to approach and exceed 20 years, it is more likely that the recipient's performance may be relatively limited. At any rate, an extended duration of deafness should not be a contraindication for cochlear implantation, but rather an indicator of the need for preimplant counseling regarding expectations. The authors also have encountered several recipients with prolonged high-frequency deafness who initially exhibit poor performance with their implant. This finding may be related to significant degeneration of spiral ganglion dendrites in the basal region of the cochlea or to deleterious changes in the central auditory system. A longer interval of implant use may be necessary before substantial benefit is attained in these recipients. For recipients who continue to struggle after several months of implant use, sound quality and speech recognition may be improved by disabling the most basal electrodes and reallocating the high-frequency inputs to more apical electrode contacts.

Advanced Age

Several published reports describe the considerable benefits of cochlear implantation for elderly adults in speech recognition and quality of life (Migirov, Taitelbaum-Swead, Drendel, Hildesheimer, & Kronenberg, 2009; Noble, Tyler, Dunn, & Bhullar, 2009); therefore, an advanced age should never dissuade a cochlear implant team from recommending implantation. However, when compared to the general adult population with implants, some recipients who have advanced age will exhibit poorer performance (Noble et al.). Therefore, more extensive counseling regarding expectations and longer appointments may be necessary. The diminished outcomes for this population may be related to the duration of deafness, changes in central auditory processing, and the neurological or cognitive status.

Internal Device Function

Although the vast majority of cochlear implant internal devices function properly, instances have been reported of compromised device integrity resulting in poor recipient performance. At some point, every manufacturer has produced an internal device with a widespread faulty component, design flaw, electrode array anomaly, or electrical defect. Clinicians should be aware of these potential issues and closely scrutinize the performance of recipients with these devices. Manufacturer representatives can provide information about the faults in past devices and the names of recipients who may have a potentially compromised device. In some cases, defects will result in complete failure of the internal device (i.e., hard device failure). In other instances, a compromised internal device may continue to provide sound for the recipient, but he or she may experience consistently poor speech recognition and/or sound quality, regression in speech recognition and/or sound quality, intermittent device function, and extraneous sounds (e.g., popping, static, crackling). The reliability data of contemporary internal devices is very high and may be found on each manufacturer's website (Advanced Bionics Corporation, 2009, April;

Cochlear Corporation, 2008, June; MED-EL Corporation, 2009, July).

If a recipient experiences a limited outcome and has a device with a suspect reliability record, the cochlear implant team should consider replacing the internal device with a new system (i.e., cochlear implant revision). Published reports and the authors' extensive anecdotal experience suggest that cochlear implant revisions frequently are successful when based on sound clinical judgment (Zeitler, Budenz, & Roland, 2009). After extensive troubleshooting and assessments, cochlear implant revision also should be considered for recipients who ought to have success with the implant (i.e., favorable preimplant history), but experience substantially poor outcomes. The decision to revise a cochlear implant is much more difficult for recipients who have any of the aforementioned factors associated with limited outcomes. Prior to the decision, the cochlear implant team should consider the recipient's intrapersonal characteristics, his or her family support, the reliability of the internal device, and the integrity of the device according to assessments conducted by programming clinician or a manufacturer representative.

Programming Adjustments for the Most Common Complaints and Complications

Prior to making programming adjustments to address recipient complaints or difficulties, the clinician needs to consider the typical periods for acclimatization following initial activation. First, sound quality and speech recognition often improve over the first few months of cochlear implant use. As a result, programming adjustments may not result in optimal sound quality during the early stages of implant use. The troubleshooting guidelines in this section may be used to improve sound quality and performance, but if the complaint persists, additional counseling may be necessary to remind the recipient that performance should improve with continued use and experience. Second, recipients usually require several days to completely adjust to any programming modifications. If a user has minor complaints about sound quality or performance immediately following a programming session, the clinician needs to use his or her clinical judgment regarding the need for additional changes to the program. The audiologist may ask the recipient to use the modified program for 7 to 10 days before additional adjustments are made. Following this period of time, most users adapt to the changes and will report better hearing than before the programming session.

Table 6–1 provides step-by-step instructions for various programming adjustments to address the most common user complaints. When a particular complaint is resolved by one of the steps, the clinician should cease the adjustments.

KEY CONCEPTS

The following key concepts were discussed in this chapter:

- Most recipients will achieve remarkable success, but others will require special programming to perform at their highest potential.
- The user's preimplant characteristics will play an important role in the postoperative implant performance.
- Appropriate and thorough preimplant counseling is absolutely necessary to help the patient set forth realistic expectations.
- Common complaints and complications often can be addressed with step-by-step modifications to stimulation levels and other programming parameters.

Table 6–1. Troubleshooting Guidelines to Address Common Recipient Complaints

Recipient Complaint	Programming Adjustments
Echo or boomy sound quality	1. Common at initial activation, allow for acclimatization. 2. Global reduction in USL; if sound too soft, return to original USL. 3. Ensure balanced loudness at USL across electrode array. 4. Reduce stimulation levels in LF channels. 5. Reduce stimulation levels in HF channels. 6. Reduce stimulation rate. 7. For CIS-type strategies, reduce gains in LF channels.* 8. For CIS-type strategies, reduce gains in HF channels.*
Ringing, pinging, or tinny sound quality	1. Ensure balanced loudness at USL across electrode array. 2. Reduction stimulation levels in HF channels. 3. Reduce stimulation rate. 4. For CIS-type strategies, reduce gains in HF channels.* 5. Sweep to locate electrodes with ringing percept; disable them. 6. Disable most basal electrode(s).
Sound is muffled, fuzzy, or not clear	1. Global increase in USL; if speech is too loud, decrease USL; if no change, return to original USL. 2. Ensure balanced loudness at USL across electrode array. 3. Increase USL in HF channels. 4. Reduce USL in LF channels. 5. Reduce stimulation rate. 6. For CIS-type strategies, increase gains in HF channels.* 7. Increase IDR. 8. Increase microphone sensitivity. 9. Global increase in threshold (T) levels. 10. Increase loudness growth function (MAPlaw) if not optimized.
Patient's own voice is too loud, but speech from others is comfortable	1. Ensure balanced loudness at USL across electrode array. 2. Global decrease in USL; if speech of others too soft, increase sensitivity, T levels, or loudness growth for low-level inputs. 3. Decrease USL in LF channels; increase USL in HF channels. 4. Global increase in gains. 5. Reduce LF gains; increase HF gains.*
Buzzing, frying, or humming sound	1. Determine ambient noise or electrical stimulation; reduce sensitivity. 2. If solved, recipient needs acclimatization to low-level sounds; if still unhappy, slightly reduce microphone sensitivity and/or IDR. 3. If not solved, adjust T levels to balance loudness at 50 percent of dynamic range. 4. Global decrease in T levels. 4. Ensure balanced loudness at USL across electrode array. 5. Global decrease in USL. 6. Decrease USL in LF channels.

Table 6–1. *continued*

Recipient Complaint	Programming Adjustments
Roaring	1. Global reduction in USL; if solved, but speech too soft, return to original USL. 2. Ensure balanced loudness at USL across electrode array. 3. Adjust T levels to balance loudness at 50 percent of dynamic range. 4. Global decrease in T levels.
Sound is hollow	1. Global reduction in USL; if sound too soft, return to original USL. 2. Ensure balanced loudness at USL across electrode array. 3. Reduction in stimulation levels at LF channels. 4. Increase in stimulation levels in HF channels. 5. Increase in stimulation levels in MF channels. 6. For CIS-type strategies, reduce gains in LF channels. 7. For CIS-type strategies, increase gains in HF or MF channels.
Overall poor sound quality/performance	1. Global increase in USL; if speech is too loud, reduce USL; use ESRT to estimate USL; if not solved, return to original USL. 2. Ensure balanced loudness at USL across electrode array. 3. Increase USL in HF channels. 4. Sweep at USL; ensure pitch percepts in expected tonotopic pattern. 5. Sweep at USL; find electrodes with poor quality/aversive percept. 6. If several months past activation, try different stimulation rates. 7. If several months past activation, try other signal coding strategies. 8. Increase PW across all channels.
Facial nerve stimulation	1. Single-channel stimulation; increase PW on channel or globally; if increased PW negatively influences loudness growth, disable electrode. 2. Stimulation in live speech mode: (a) sweep at USL to find problem channels; (b) may increase maximum USL permissible to elicit facial stimulation; (c) disable 2–3 electrodes a time in live speech mode to find problem; (d) increase PW or disable problem electrodes. 3. If stimulation still exists with 25 percent electrodes disabled: change the electrode coupling mode (i.e., monopolar or bipolar).
Discomfort, pain, nonauditory percept, such as tinnitus or tactile sensation	1. Measure ESRT to see whether USL is too high. 2. Sweep at USL; find suspect channels, increase PW, remeasure stimulation levels; if not solved, disable electrodes. 3. Disable 2–3 electrodes a time in live speech mode to find problem; increase PW or disable problem electrodes. 4. If problem across several electrodes, increase PW for all electrodes. 5. Change electrode coupling mode (i.e., monopolar or bipolar). 5. Decrease stimulation rate; high rate may cause tinnitus/vibration. 6. Change signal coding strategy.

Notes. *should not be done for *n*-of-*m* coding strategies; IDR = input dynamic range; HF = high-frequency; LF = low-frequency; MF = mid-frequency; PW = pulse width; USL = upper stimulation levels

||| 7 |||

Hearing Assistance Technology (HAT) and Cochlear Implants

Adults and children who use cochlear implants often achieve good open-set speech perception in quiet listening situations; however, they will experience significant difficulty understanding speech in the presence of background noise. In fact, when compared to average performance in quiet, speech perception in noise is significantly poorer by approximately 40% (Fetterman & Domico, 2002; Firzst et al., 2004; Schafer & Thibodeau, 2004). Similar performance detriments are found when comparing average scores in noise of people with cochlear implants and normal-hearing peers. The use of HAT, such as personal frequency modulated (FM) systems, addresses these listening difficulties in noise by directing the signal from the primary talker straight to the listener's ear.

HAT provides significant improvements in speech recognition in noise for adults and children ranging from 29 to 44% when compared to performance with the cochlear implant alone (Schafer & Thibodeau, 2004; Wolfe & Schafer, 2008). Furthermore, when using HAT adults report improved clarity, ease of listening, and sound quality when communicating in small and large groups.

The chapter introduces personal wireless devices for improving speech perception in noise and discusses programming considerations for coupling sound processors to HAT. These sections are followed by an overview of devices for improving telephone conversations.

BASIC DESCRIPTION OF PERSONAL SYSTEMS

Two types of personal systems may be used with cochlear implants: (1) devices using FM or infrared (light) transmission or (2) induction loop systems utilizing electromagnetic transmission (i.e., telecoil). When using FM systems, the talker wears a transmitter and microphone, and the listener uses a device that plugs directly into the cochlear implant sound processor. A personal, ear-level or body-worn receiver decodes the FM or infrared signal, converts it to an electrical signal, and sends it through the sound processor. Personal receivers are connected to the sound processor using a manufacturer-specific battery cover, cable, adaptor, or earhook.

Induction loop receivers may be used only when the recipient has an active telecoil in his or her sound processor (i.e., Auria, Harmony, ESPrit 3G, Freedom, CP810, OPUS 2). The transmitter sends the speech signal via infrared or FM transmission to an induction receiver. The electrical signal from the receiver is converted to an electromagnetic signal and sent through a loop of wire that is placed around the listener's neck (i.e., neckloop) or around the room. The listener's active telecoil detects the electromagnetic signal and converts it back into an electrical signal, which then is processed by the cochlear implant. When an induction loop is placed around a room, no specialized equipment is required. Conversely, when using a neckloop, a specialized body-worn induction receiver must be used.

OPTIMAL SYSTEMS FOR USE WITH A COCHLEAR IMPLANT

The only published studies available on HAT and cochlear implants are related to performance with FM technology. To the authors' knowledge, no studies have examined the benefits of infrared technology or induction loop arrangements for users of cochlear implants.

According to a recent meta-analysis—the strongest level of evidence according to the American Speech-Language-Hearing Association (2004)—personal FM systems provide the best speech recognition in noise when compared to sound-field (i.e., loudspeaker) FM systems (Schafer & Kleineck, in press). The personal system provided a 38% improvement over the cochlear implant alone, as compared to the 17% and 4% improvements from the two soundfield systems, respectively. Although no studies have been published on the benefits of induction loop systems for people with cochlear implants, patient reports suggest that these systems provide similar benefits as those achieved with personal FM systems.

DESCRIPTION AND PROGRAMMING FOR PERSONAL HAT AND COCHLEAR IMPLANTS

FM Transmitters

Contemporary FM transmitters—cell-phone-sized, rechargeable devices that are worn on a belt or lavaliere—are used for any population (e.g., hearing aid, normal hearing). Four commonly used FM transmitters are shown in Figure 7–1. Each of these transmitters offers various options for the listener including microphone style (Figure 7–2), directionality for the microphone, multichannel

capabilities, and programmability. These transmitters may be used with FM or induction loop receivers.

Programmable FM transmitters offer the audiologist a great deal of flexibility when determining the optimal settings for an adult or child with a cochlear implant. Programming options include selection of one or more transmitting channels, wireless programming of the FM receiver (e.g., channel, FM gain), DataLogging (i.e., storing noise level), creation of wireless team-teaching connections (i.e., combined signal from more than one talker at a time), evaluation of transmitter/receiver function, monitoring of classroom noise, and help with channel selection in an environment to avoid interference. Most transmitters also have an auxiliary input port to allow for connection to audio sources including televisions, computers, DVD players, and tape players. One transmitter has Bluetooth technology (Phonak SmarkLink), which may be used with Bluetooth compatible phones.

FM and Induction Loop Receivers

Two contemporary miniaturized FM receivers are shown in Figure 7–3. As outlined in Table 7–1 and shown in Figure 7–4, these miniaturized receivers connect to body-worn and ear-level cochlear implant speech processors in one of four ways: (1) specialized receiver adaptors plus cables, (2) FM adaptor, (3) FM earhook, and (4) design integration/direct connect.

Some of the programmable options on the Amigo R1/R2 receivers include 0 to 30 dB of programmable gain (i.e., FM advantage over input from implant sound processor), multichannel capability, programmable default channel, programmable switch, sleep mode, manual channel seek button, tamper resistant switches, and wireless programmability. Options on the Phonak MLxi include multichannel capability, adaptive FM advantage (i.e., Dynamic FM when used with the inspiro transmitter), FM advantage adjustment, and sleep/stand-by mode. Dynamic FM is available when using the Phonak inspiro transmitter and companion receiver (i.e., MLxi). This technology automatically adjusts the gain of the FM receiver depending on the noise level in the environment.

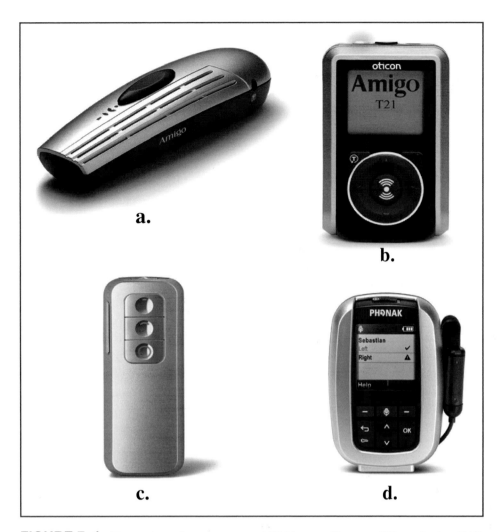

FIGURE 7–1. Examples of contemporary FM transmitters: **a.** Oticon Amigo T10; **b.** Oticon Amigo T21; **c.** Phonak SmartLink SX; **d.** Phonak inspiro. Courtesy of Oticon Inc. and Phonak.

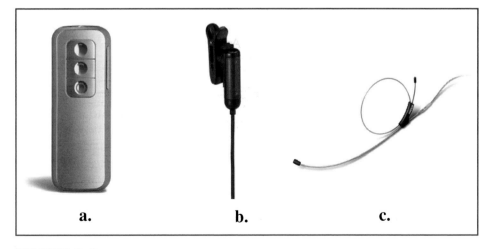

FIGURE 7–2. Examples of FM transmitter microphones: **a.** Phonak SmartLink SX integrated microphones; **b.** Phonak iLapel microphone; **c.** Phonak iBoom microphone (cheek). Courtesy of Phonak.

When the noise level exceeds 57 dB SPL, the gain of the receiver is increased automatically (from a default +10 gain) to maintain a favorable signal-to-noise ratio at the listener's ear. Several previous generations of Phonak receivers (e.g., Micro MLxS, and MLxS) also offered multichannel capability, FM advantage adjustment, soft squelch (turns off receiver when transmitter off), and sleep mode. Given the fact that FM system technology continues to evolve and change, cochlear implant and FM system manufacturers recognize the need for audiologist, teacher, and parent education. As such, most manufacturers provide online training and support, knowledgeable representatives, and step-by-step guides to aid the audiologist, and sometimes teachers and parents, with ordering appropriate equipment, procedures for connecting to a cochlear implant, information about using FM systems, and instructions for troubleshooting problems.

Two examples of contemporary induction loop receivers with built-in neckloops are provided in Figure 7–5. The Phonak MyLink is a multichannel, rechargeable FM receiver that includes

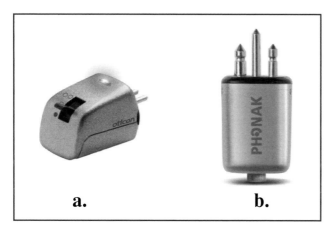

a.   **b.**

FIGURE 7–3. Examples of two contemporary FM receivers: **a.** Oticon Amigo; **b.** Phonak MLxi. Courtesy of Oticon Inc. and Phonak.

Table 7–1. Equipment for Connecting Oticon and Phonak Frequency Modulated (FM) Receivers to Cochlear Implant (CI) Sound Processors

Type of Connection	Examples of Equipment	Used with Cochlear Implant Sound Processors
Specialized Receiver Adaptors with Cables	• Oticon Amigo FM-CI adaptor plus processor-specific cord[1] • Phonak MicroLink CI-S adaptor plus processor specific-cord[2]	• All body-worn processors • Most all older ear-level processors • Amigo FM-CI adaptor used for Cochlear Freedom BTE
FM Adaptor	• ESPrit 3G MicroLink Adaptor[1,2]	• Cochlear ESPrit 3G
FM Earhook	• Advanced Bionics iConnect earhook[1,2] • Advanced Bionics Auxillary Audio Earhook with cable[1,2,3]	• Advanced Bionics Harmony & Auria processors • Advanced Bionics CII & Platinum BTE processors
Design Integration & Direct Connect	• *Integration:* MicroLink Freedom FM (FM built into battery pack) • *Direct Connect:* Receivers[1,2] plugged straight to processor	• Cochlear Freedom BTE • Freedom Body-Worn, MED-EL OPUS 2 with FM battery pack • CP810 with FM Euro (not released yet)

Notes. [1]Equipment may be connected to Oticon Amigo R1 and R2 receivers; [2]equipment may be connected to Phonak MicroMLxS, MLxS, & MLxi receivers; [3]also requires the use of a specialized receiver adaptor with cables; BTE = behind the ear.

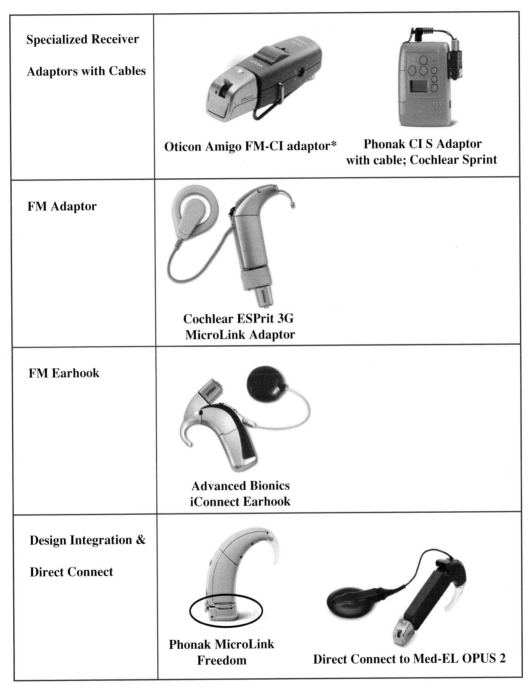

Specialized Receiver Adaptors with Cables	Oticon Amigo FM-CI adaptor*	Phonak CI S Adaptor with cable; Cochlear Sprint
FM Adaptor	Cochlear ESPrit 3G MicroLink Adaptor	
FM Earhook	Advanced Bionics iConnect Earhook	
Design Integration & Direct Connect	Phonak MicroLink Freedom	Direct Connect to Med-EL OPUS 2

FIGURE 7–4. Examples of each type of connection between the cochlear implant sound processor and personal FM system. *Note:* * = cable not shown. Courtesy of Oticon Inc. and Phonak.

several characteristics including a noise blocker to reduce the input from the FM system when in a quiet environment, a sleep mode to reduce the input from the FM transmitter when it is not in use (i.e., avoid hissing noise), wireless synchroniza-tion, and an input port for regular headphones to allow for troubleshooting from a normal-hearing listener. The Oticon Arc is also a multichannel, rechargeable FM receiver with sleep mode, wireless synchronization, wireless programming, adjustable

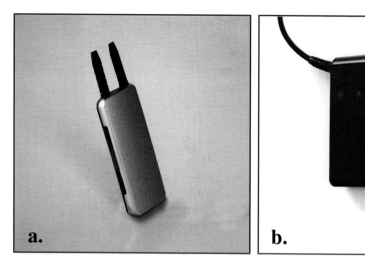

FIGURE 7–5. Two examples of contemporary induction neckloop receivers: **a.** Phonak MyLink; **b.** Oticon Arc. Courtesy of Oticon Inc. and Phonak.

receiver gain, tamper resistant switch, channel seek function, and status indicator. Both of these devices allow for connection to auxiliary input from other audio sources including computers, televisions, and CD players.

At the time of this writing, the induction loop FM receiver is the primary HAT option for the CP810 sound processor. In the near future, Cochlear Corporation plans to release a three-port Euro plug adaptor that will connect directly to the accessory port of the processor. It will allow for the automatic detection of and coupling of personal FM receivers to the sound processor. As mentioned in Chapter 1, the CP810 sound processor has an automatic telecoil, which utilizes a patented algorithm to automatically engage to speech-like electromagnetic signals from induction loops. This feature is unique in the hearing industry, as the typical automatic telecoils found in hearing aids will activate to telephones, but not to induction neckloops.

Programming Considerations for FM Receivers and Sound Processors

FM-Receiver Programming

On the FM receiver, the gain may be adjusted to alter the relationship of the signals from the FM system and processor microphones. For the Oticon Amigo R1/R2 and Phonak MLxi, Micro MLxS, and MLxS miniaturized receivers, a 30-dB range of gain is offered. A higher gain setting, such as +15 to +20, provides greater advantage for the signal from the FM system relative to the input from the sound processor microphone.

Previous research suggests that higher gain settings allow for significantly better speech perception in noise than lower gain settings (Schafer, Wolfe, Lawless, & Stout, 2009; Wolfe & Schafer, 2008). According to the results of these studies, optimal performance and comfort for nine adults and five children using Advanced Bionics implants was achieved with +14 and +16 receiver-gain settings. Conversely, increased receiver-gain settings did provide better performance for eight users of Cochlear Corporation sound processors. Differences in performance between the two manufacturer groups were likely related to sound processor settings, which are discussed in the following section. No studies have been conducted on the effects of receiver gain for users of MED-EL cochlear implants, but similar results are expected as those obtained with other devices.

Recent research suggests that Dynamic FM results in significantly better speech recognition in noise than traditional FM systems set to +10 dB gain for users of Advanced Bionics devices (Wolfe et al., 2009). In the initial experiment, users of

Cochlear Corporation Freedom did not show significant benefit from either type of FM system. However, when a certain parameter in the Freedom programming was adjusted (i.e., Autosensitivity), speech recognition results were similar to those using Advanced Bionics implants. According to the results of this study, Dynamic FM may provide even greater benefit to users of cochlear implants than traditional FM systems.

Sound Processor Programming and HAT

Several parameters in sound processor programming may significantly influence performance with a personal FM system including audio-mixing ratio, input dynamic range (IDR), and sensitivity.

Audio-Mixing Ratios. Similar to FM gain, audio-mixing ratios determine the relationship or ratio between the inputs from the sound processor and the FM transmitter microphones. Although this discussion is focused on FM systems, some of the ratios are applicable to telecoil settings for any auxiliary-audio device (e.g., iPod; MP3 player) that is electrically coupled to the sound processor.

The Auria and Harmony Advanced Bionics sound processors may be programmed with five fixed audio-mixing ratios: (1) 30/70, processor microphone attenuated by 10 dB; (2) 50/50, equal emphasis, (3) auxiliary only attenuated, processor microphone attenuated by 20 dB; (4) auxiliary only, no processor microphone; and (5) microphone only, no auxiliary input. The 50/50 is the default setting, but the 30/70 and the 50/50 ratios are commonly used. Cochlear Corporation CP810 and Freedom processors allow for four mixing ratios including a (1) 1:1-equal emphasis, (2) 2:1-processor microphone attenuated by 6 dB, (3) 3:1-processor microphone attenuated by 9.5 dB, and (4) 10:1-processor microphone attenuated by 20 dB. In the CP810, the mixing ratios are adjusted with the CR110 wireless remote control, while mixing ratios for the Freedom are set in the programming software.

According to previous research on 12 adults using Advanced Bionics sound processors and FM receivers, no significant differences in speech perception or subjective benefit exist between a 30/70 and 50/50 audio-mixing ratio (Wolfe &

Schafer, 2008). However, when attempting to hear low-level speech in quiet that was directed to the sound processor (i.e., not to the FM transmitter), the adults performed significantly poorer when using the 30/70 mixing ratio. Preliminary data collected in the authors' laboratories (not in reference list) shows similar results for adults using Cochlear Corporation Freedom sound processors when comparing the 3:1 and 1:1 ratios. Therefore, to ensure audibility of FM and environmental signals, a 50/50 or 1:1 mixing ratio is recommended for users of Auria and CP810/Freedom processors, respectively.

The previous generation Cochlear Corporation ESPrit 3G processor does not have pre-set mixing ratios. Instead, the audio-mixing ratio is determined by the sensitivity setting on the sound processor. When the ESPrit 3G knob is programmed for sensitivity, a lower sensitivity setting on the knob will provide more FM input, while a higher knob setting will provide more input from the sound processor. When the knob is set for volume, the sensitivity level is fixed and predetermined in the programming software. No published research exists on the optimal sensitivity setting for the processor when using a personal FM receiver; however, some unpublished data does support the theory that lower sensitivity settings may result in better speech recognition in noise (Aaron, Sonneveldt, Arcaroli, & Holstad, 2003). In addition, previous studies show substantial FM benefit for adults and children with typical processor sensitivity settings (Schafer & Thibodeau, 2003 Schafer et al., 2009).

MED-EL Tempo+, OPUS 1, and OPUS 2 sound processors do not offer various mixing ratios for FM systems. A 1:1 audio-mixing ratio is enabled automatically. If the user desires an FM-only setting, the sensitivity on the sound processor knob may be turned to the off position (i.e., 11:00). No published data demonstrates the benefits of personal FM systems for users of MED-EL cochlear implants, but according to anecdotal reports (not in reference list) these users obtain FM benefit.

Input Dynamic Range (IDR). As discussed in the section on FM-receiver gain, findings from two studies revealed greater FM benefit for users of Advanced Bionics versus Cochlear Corporation processors (Schafer et al., 2007; Wolfe et al., 2009). The differences between the two processor groups likely are related to the upper range of the IDR settings in the sound processor. The IDR is the range of acoustic-input levels (i.e., 30 to 60 dB) that are coded by the sound processor within the user's electrical dynamic range. Signal levels that exceed the upper end of the IDR are subjected to high-level compression, and low-level signals below the IDR are not processed and are likely inaudible to the listener.

Advanced Bionics implants have a default IDR of 60 dB SPL. As such, inputs ranging from 25 to 85 dB SPL typically are mapped into the person's electrical dynamic range. The goal of this wide IDR is to provide audibility for low-level inputs, while avoiding the negative effects of high-level environmental noise. MED-EL sound processors use a similar wide IDR of approximately 55 dB SPL. In contrast, Cochlear Corporation implants use a narrower default IDR of 30 dB SPL for ESPrit 3G processors and 40 dB SPL for Freedom sound processors. As a result, inputs of 35 to 65 dB SPL and 25 to 65 dB SPL will be mapped for users of ESPrit 3G and Freedom processors, respectively. The goal of a narrower IDR is to code continuously the rapid fluctuations in speech into the electrical dynamic range.

The IDR may influence the signal from the FM system for two reasons: (1) typical signals from an FM system are often at a higher intensity (i.e., 75 dB SPL), and (2) the IDR influences the signals coded at the upper end of the dynamic range. When using a narrow IDR (i.e., Cochlear Corporation) with an upper end of 65 dB SPL, the signal from the FM system likely will be compressed. Furthermore, any increases in FM-receiver gain will not be coded by the implant or perceived by the listener. In other words, speech recognition in noise with an FM-receiver gain of +10 dB would produce similar performance as FM receivers programmed for +14 or +16 gain. Compression of the FM signal is less probable for users of Advanced Bionics implants because the upper end of the IDR is 85 dB SPL, which allows for processor coding and user perception of increases in receiver gain. Further research is necessary to determine an ideal IDR for users of cochlear implants cou-

pled to personal FM systems. At this time, the IDR parameter is not adjusted for FM use.

Processor Sensitivity. The effects of a narrow IDR may be addressed by changes to the third parameter, microphone sensitivity. The sensitivity determines the gain for inputs from the sound processor microphone (i.e., softest sound that will be picked up by the microphone). When sensitivity is increased from the default setting, lower intensity sounds from a distance will be mapped into the user's electrical dynamic range. A decrease to the sensitivity, however, will reduce the user's ability to hear soft and distant speech, which may improve hearing in background noise. In addition, some evidence shows that lower sensitivity settings provide significantly better speech recognition in noise for users of Cochlear Corporation implants than higher sensitivity settings when using an FM system (Aaron et al., 2003).

While reductions to sensitivity may increase the audibility of the FM system, it also may influence negatively the user's ability to hear environmental sounds. Therefore, it is important to find a good balance between the two signals, which may require behavioral testing or a good reporter (i.e., older child or adult). For younger children, access to the sensitivity may be disabled on the sound processor and fixed in the sound processor programming. When this is the case, it is best to leave the sensitivity at the typical user setting, even when an FM system is in use.

The effect of the sensitivity control varies between the CP810 and Freedom sound processors. For the Freedom processor, the sensitivity setting affects only the signal from the sound processor microphone with no attenuation provided to the FM signal. As a result, lower sensitivity settings will provide greater emphasis on the FM signal. However, the high-level signal from the FM system will be subjected to compression at the input of the Freedom processor. In contrast, the sensitivity setting for the CP810 processor affects the gain applied to the signals from both the sound processor microphone and the FM system. Therefore, lower sensitivity settings prevent both signals from being subjected to compression. Because the FM input should be higher than the ambient noise level in many instances, the FM advantage should be preserved. Also, at lower sensitivity settings, an increase in FM receiver gain provided through manual adjustments or with Dynamic FM should be more beneficial to the user because the increased strength of the FM signal is not compressed at the input of the sound processor. Similarly, MED-EL processors have a fixed 1:1 audio-mixing ratio. Changes to sensitivity influence only the signal at the processor microphone; therefore, a reduction to sensitivity may result in greater emphasis for the FM signal. Reducing the sound processor sensitivity to zero on the Freedom and to the off position on MED-EL devices will deactivate the processor microphone and result in an FM-only condition.

Another programmable option for users of Cochlear Corporation implants is an input-preprocessing feature known as Autosensitivity (ASC). This optional setting automatically reduces the sensitivity of the processor microphone according to the noise level in the environment and the signal-to-noise ratio at the microphone. The goal of ASC is for the peaks of speech to exceed the long-term-average spectrum of the noise by at least 15 dB when the noise level in the environment exceeds 57 dB SPL.

According to previous research, the use of ASC will improve significantly speech-recognition performance in noise with FM relative to a condition with no ASC (Wolfe et al., 2009). This also should be true for the CP810 sound processor. In addition, when the ASC parameter was enabled, speech recognition with Dynamic FM was no longer significantly different between users of Advanced Bionics and Cochlear Corporation implants. This occurred because ASC reduces the effects of the narrow IDR for users of Cochlear Corporation implants, and it allows for improved speech recognition performance in noise with increases to receiver gain. Results of another condition in this study revealed that use of ASC also improved performance when the speech signal was presented to the processor microphone with the FM transmitter muted. In summary, this research supports the use of ASC for users of Cochlear Corporation implants in noise with and without the use of a personal FM system.

Fitting Procedures for Personal FM Systems

Given the improved compatibility of personal FM systems and sound processors, connecting the two devices is fairly simple. To aid with these connections, cochlear implant and FM system manufacturers offer step-by-step guides, online and in print, as well as onsite and phone support from representatives. As such, the majority of this section focuses on fitting procedures following the successful connection of a personal FM system to a cochlear implant. However, an introduction to connecting the devices is provided.

In general, as a first step to connecting the devices, the FM system receiver, FM transmitter, and sound processor are turned off. Second, the FM receiver is connected to the sound processor with the appropriate adaptor, cable, or earhook. Then, for most systems, the speech processor is turned on, followed by activation of the FM receiver and transmitter. Finally, a listener with normal-hearing sensitivity performs a listening check after this connection is made, which is described in the following section on monitoring and troubleshooting.

At the time of the fitting, the adult or older child should be tested in a quiet and noise condition with and without the FM system. The speech-recognition measure needs to have multiple lists that are equivalently difficult in the type of noise that will be used (i.e., multitalker babble). In addition, the speech and noise need to be recorded on different channels so that they may be presented from spatially separated loudspeakers.

When percent-correct scoring is used, the test material needs to be challenging enough, in quiet and in noise, to avoid ceiling effects (i.e., 100% correct). Adaptive test measures (i.e., Hearing in Noise Test; Nilsson, Soli, & Sullivan, 1994) may be used; however, it may be best if the noise adapts while the speech remains at a constant intensity (i.e., 60 dBA). This accounts for effects of transmitter compression, which will occur during testing because the speech is presented at a typical intensity (i.e., 70 dB SPL at the location of transmitter).

Speech-recognition testing may be conducted in a soundproof booth or in a classroom setting for students. The single-coned speech loudspeaker should be placed at zero degrees azimuth and at least 3 feet from the listener. One or more noise loudspeakers should be spatially separated from the signal loudspeaker by at least 30 degrees. When the FM system is in use, the microphone of the FM transmitter should be placed 3 (boom microphones) to 6 (lapel microphones) inches from the center of the single-coned loudspeaker to replicate the distance of the microphone from the talker's mouth.

The results of the two speech-recognition conditions in quiet ought to show negligible differences between the FM and no-FM conditions or slightly better performance in the FM condition. Conversely, speech recognition in noise should be considerably better in the FM condition when compared to the no-FM condition. Significance between conditions may be determined through the use of 95% confidence intervals, which often are provided in the user manual of the test material. If ceiling effects (i.e., 100% correct) occur in any conditions, the signal or noise levels may be adjusted to allow for a more challenging testing situation and for additional headroom for condition comparisons. When these results do not occur, the audiologist may consider adjusting the gain of the FM receiver, audio-mixing ratio, or sensitivity of the sound processor. These conditions then can be repeated until the desired results are obtained.

For younger children and people with cognitive deficits, it is difficult to perform usual speech-recognition measures. Instead, the parent or caregiver needs to monitor the functioning of the cochlear implant and FM device once to twice a day using procedures described in the following section on troubleshooting.

Some manufacturers and professionals do not recommend FM systems for young children; however, no evidence suggests that a well-fit and monitored FM system will be detrimental to a child's speech and language development. On the contrary, a large body of research supports the use of FM systems for adults and children with cochlear implants for improving speech recognition in quiet and noisy situations. These improvements are likely to aid in speech and language development. In the authors' opinion, the inability of the child to report difficulties with the FM device should not

be a reason for nonuse, as being a good reporter is not a requirement for receiving a cochlear implant. The following section provides several avenues for monitoring and troubleshooting FM and implant devices.

Monitoring and Troubleshooting Personal FM Systems for Cochlear Implants

Troubleshooting of personal FM systems may be a challenge for people with normal-hearing sensitivity; nonetheless, with the correct equipment, the audiologist has numerous ways to verify functioning of the cochlear implant speech processor and FM receiver separately. To determine proper functioning of the sound processor, the audiologist or parent may use a coil-check wand, transmission symbols or lights on the processor, and monitor earphones. These earphones allow a person with normal-hearing sensitivity to listen to acoustic signals presented to the sound processor microphone.

The signal from the FM system may be verified by conducting a behavioral listening check or by using more objective techniques, which include listening to the signal from an amplifier speaker, extra hearing aid with an audio shoe, headset checker, or sound processor monitor earphones. When conducting a behavioral listening check, the child is asked to repeat words or sounds that he or she hears as a person speaks into the transmitter microphone. This technique verifies functional performance of the FM system and allows the audiologist to determine function of a processed signal through the cochlear implant. However, these procedures may not be possible for young children or patients with cognitive delays or disorders.

In addition to a behavioral check, the audiologist should verify the signal through some type of amplifier. Several options are available for listening to the signal from the FM system alone. First, when using the Oticon CI-FM Adaptor or Phonak MicroLink CI S coupled to a miniaturized FM receiver, the signal may be verified by speaking into the transmitter microphone and listening to the output from the FM receiver through an amplifier. Amplifiers may include an inexpensive, small speaker with an ⅛-inch input (e.g., Radio Shack Mini Audio Amplifier) or an extra hearing aid with the appropriate FM audio shoe (approximately $30–50). Another amplifier option is a Headset Checker from Phonak that allows for direct connection of a miniaturized FM receiver to headphones. The normal-hearing listener can verify acoustic signals from the FM receiver through the earphones while speaking into the transmitter microphone.

The best way to check the FM signal while connected to a sound processor is with monitor earphones, which are available for current and previous generation sound processors from Cochlear Corporation. The monitor earphones are plugged directly into the speech processor and allow the audiologist or parent to listen to the combined signals from the speech processor microphone and from the FM transmitter microphone. When checking the sound processor, the sensitivity may be reduced or turned all the way down to verify the FM signal. Conversely, when verifying the signal from the processor microphone, the FM transmitter may be muted, and the sensitivity of the sound processor may be increased. The signal from the monitor earphones is not processed all the way through the cochlear implant internal device; however, they allow for verification of the signal from the microphone just prior to entering the speech processor.

HAT TO IMPROVE TELEPHONE CONVERSATIONS

In general, two options exist for improving telephone conversations over what is achieved with the sound processor alone. These options include (1) direct-audio input of the signal from the phone to the processor and (2) transmission of the signal from the phone to the processor with a telecoil. As expected, direct-audio input requires a direct-electrical connection between the phone and the sound processor. Each manufacturer provides a special cord for connecting sound processors to

land-line phones. The telecoil option, however, may allow for a wireless connection between a land-line or cell phone and a sound processor. The following two sections introduce the standard use of telecoils, programming considerations, and telecoil accessories for cochlear implants.

Telecoils

The general procedures for using a telecoil are similar across cochlear implant manufacturers. The first step is to obtain a regular land-line telephone or telecoil-compatible cell phone. All cell phone manufacturers make telecoil compatible phones. In fact, as of 2006, the Federal Communications Commission requires that all cell phone providers have at least two highly rated telecoil compatible phones. After the processor is set to the telecoil setting, or the telecoil adaptor is connected, the telephone conversation may begin. During the conversation, the person may need to adjust the location of the telephone receiver relative to the telecoil (i.e., above or behind the sound processor) to obtain the best orientation and signal from the phone receiver.

Manufacturer-Specific Information

As previously mentioned, all contemporary sound processors have built-in telecoils. In addition, several previous generation (i.e., Tempo, Auria) or contemporary (i.e., Harmony) sound processors have an external telecoil adaptor that plugs directly into the sound processor. The telecoil options discussed in this section also are applicable to the use of induction-loop HAT with a room loop or neckloop via FM or infrared technology. In fact, several of the external devices, as described in the following section, use an induction neckloop to send the signal from the phone to the sound processor.

The Advanced Bionics Harmony has a built-in telecoil and two telecoil settings the audiologist may select from in the programming software (i.e., 50/50, 30/70). Through programming, the audiologist needs to make the telecoil active and its function accessible in one of the switch positions on the sound processor. Advanced Bionics also offers a telecoil adaptor that may be plugged into the Direct Connect Earhook. Users of Harmony processors may consider using the telecoil adaptor when no program is available for the built-in telecoil or when the user does not desire to use a program position for the built-in telecoil. The previous generation processor, the Auria, does not have a built-in telecoil, but a Telecoil Adaptor may be connected to the processor via the Direct Connect Earhook and cable.

The Cochlear Corporation CP810, Freedom, and ESPrit 3G processors also have a built-in telecoil. In fact, the CP810 telecoil can be accessed manually via a push-button on the sound processor or CR110 wireless remote control, or it can be set to automatically engage to telephone or neckloop signals. On the Freedom processor, telecoil access may be placed in one of the program slots, and similar to the Harmony, the same audio-mixing ratios are available as those for FM use. The ESPrit 3G has a telecoil switch at the bottom of the processor.

The MED-EL OPUS 2 has a FineTuner remote control, which allows the user to select from three signal-source settings: microphone only, telecoil only, or microphone plus telecoil (1:1 ratio). The previous generation sound processor for MED-EL, the Tempo+, has a TeleMic accessory that consists of an external telecoil plus an external microphone to improve listening in noisy situations. The TeleMic has a three-position switch: off, telecoil, and external microphone. In all three positions, the sound processor microphone remains active, but the input is slightly reduced. When using the phone, the TeleMic should be held against the receiver of the land-line phone.

Telecoil Accessories

Several other telecoil accessories may be coupled to most sound processors with specialized cables. These products are sold by many HAT vendors. The newest type of system utilizes Bluetooth technology along with a neckloop (e.g., MaxIT Bluetooth Cellphone Neckloop; Starkey ELI Neck-

loop) or headset (e.g., Motorola HS850 Bluetooth Headset). To use either device, the user needs a cell phone with Bluetooth capabilities as well as an active built-in telecoil or telecoil adaptor. The speech signal from the telephone is sent via Bluetooth to the receiver, which is worn by the listener. The receiver decodes the signal and sends it through the neckloop or headset. Finally, the telecoil that is built-in or connected to the sound processor detects and decodes the electromagnetic signal from the neckloop/headset and sends it through the processor. These devices also include a microphone, allowing the user to have hands-free conversations.

The second device, a phone neckloop, functions in the exact same manner as the Bluetooth device, but a wired connection exists to the cell or land-line phone. The neckloop will plug into a 2.5- or 3.5-mm jack on the phone. In addition to the neckloop, some devices have a microphone to allow for two-way conversations (i.e., listening and speaking), and others do not have the microphone (i.e. audio-only neckloops).

Another telecoil accessory, the silhouette, is a lightweight, wafer-thin earpiece that creates an induction connection from the cell or land-line phone to the sound processor. It functions similarly to neckloops whereby the silhouette, which is electrically connected to land-line or cell phones, transmits electromagnetic information to the sound processor telecoil.

SUMMARY OF HAT FOR COCHLEAR IMPLANTS

Despite the advances in cochlear implant technology, users continue to experience difficulties with speech perception in noise and over the telephone. However, as discussed in this chapter, several types of HAT are available to improve speech recognition in noise and telephone conversations of people with cochlear implants. When considering types of HAT for speech recognition, evidence-based research supports the use of personal FM systems that electrically couple to sound processors. When the FM system is successfully connected to the sound processor, several programming parameters may need adjusting including the gain of the FM receiver and audio-mixing ratios, IDR, and sensitivity of the sound processor. These parameters have a significant influence on speech recognition in quiet and in noise; therefore, the audiologist wants to use the most up-to-date research and individualized testing to determine the optimal settings for a patient.

HAT for improving telephone conversations may involve direct-audio input of the signal from the phone to the sound processor or use of a telecoil that is built-in or plugged into the sound processor. Through electromagnetic transmission, the telecoil allows the user to hear land-line or telecoil-compatible cell phone conversations through the implant. Several telecoil accessories also are available to transmit the sound from a land-line or cell phone through the use of electromagnetic (i.e., neckloop or silhouette) or Bluetooth transmission. Furthermore, HAT may offer particular improvement in telephone performance for bilateral cochlear implant recipients, as it may allow these users to listen to telephone output with both cochlear implants simultaneously.

KEY CONCEPTS

The reader should understand how to use HAT with cochlear implants and understand the following key concepts:

- Speech perception in noise of people using unilateral or bilateral cochlear implants is improved significantly when using personal HAT, such as an FM system, relative to performance with an implant alone.
- The most commonly used personal HAT for people with cochlear implants is FM systems and induction loop systems.
- There are several manufacturer-specific programming considerations for sound processors when coupling to personal HAT.
- The primary way to improve telephone conversations with a cochlear implant is through the use of a telecoil, which may require special programming or adaptors for the sound processor.

References

Aaron, R., Sonneveldt, V., Arcaroli, J., & Holstad, B. (2003). Optimizing microphone sensitivity settings of pediatric Nucleus 24 cochlear implant patients using Phonak MicroLink CI+ FM system. Poster presented at ACCESS: Achieving Clear Communications Employing Sound Solutions: Proceedings of the First International Conference, Chicago, IL. *Acoustical Society of America, 100*(4), 2393–2414.

Advanced Bionics Corporation. (2003). New Methodology for Fitting Cochlear Implants. Retrieved October 19, 2009, from http://www.advancedbionics.com/For_Professionals/Library/Technical_Reports.cfm?langid=1

Advanced Bionics Corporation. (2009, March). *HiRes with Fidelity 120® Clinical Results.* Retrieved October 12, 2009, from http://www.advancedbionics.com/UserFiles/File/3-01009-A_HiRes120_Clinical%20Results%28Mar_05%29.pdf

Advanced Bionics Corporation. (2009, April). *Harmony HiResolution Bionic Ear System: Number One in System Reliability and Durability-Guaranteed.* Retrieved October 8, 2009, from http://www.advancedbionics.com/UserFiles/File/3-01131A_ConsumerReliability_Report-FNL.pdf

American Speech-Language-Hearing Association. (2004). *Evidence-based practice in communication disorders: An introduction* [Technical Report].

Anderson, I., Baumgartner, W. D., Boheim, K., Nahler, A., Arnoldner, C., & D'Haese, P. (2006). Telephone use: What benefit do cochlear implant users receive? *International Journal of Audiology, 45*(8), 446–453.

Arnoldner, C., Baumgartner, W. D., Gstoettner, W., Egelierler, B., Czerny, C., Steiner, E., & Hamzavi, J. (2004). Audiological performance after cochlear implantation in children with inner ear malformations. *International Journal of Pediatric Otorhinolaryngology, 68*(4), 457–467.

Arnolder, C., Riss, D., Brunner, M., Durisin, M., Baumgartner, W. D., & Hamzavi, J. S. (2007). Speech and music perception with the new fine structure speech coding strategy: preliminary results. *Acta Otolaryngologica, 127*(12), 1298–1303.

Arora, K., Dawson. P., Dowell, R., & Vandali. A. (2009). Electrical stimulation rate effects on speech perception in cochlear implants. *International Journal of Audiology, 48*(8), 561–567.

Balkany, T., Hodges, A., Menapace, C., Hazard, L., Driscoll, C., Gantz, B., . . . Payne, S. (2007). Nucleus Freedom North American clinical trial. *Otolaryngology Head and Neck Surgery, 136*(5), 757–762.

Battmer, R. D., Laszig, R., & Lehnhardt, E. (1990). Electrically elicited stapedius reflex in cochlear implant patients. *Ear and Hearing, 11*(5), 370–374.

Baudhuin, J., Cadieux, J., Reeder, R. M., Kettel, J., Firszt, J. B. (2009, June). *Optimization of speech processor fitting in children.* Presented at the 12th Symposium on Cochlear Implants in Children, Seattle, WA.

Bent III, J. P., Chute, P., & Parisier, S. C. (1999). Cochlear implantation in children with enlarged vestibular aqueducts. *Laryngoscope, 109*(7 Pt 1), 1019–1022.

Beynon, A. J., Snik, A. F., & van den Broek, P. (2003). Comparison of different speech coding strategies using a disability-based inventory and speech perception tests in quiet and in noise. *Otology and Neurotology, 24*(3), 392–396.

Bresnihan, M., Norman, G., Scott, F., & Viani, L. (2001). Measurement of comfort levels by means of electrical stapedial reflex in children. *Archives of Otolaryngology–Head & Neck Surgery, 127*(8), 963–966.

Brickley, G., Boyd, P., Wyllie, F., O'Driscoll, M., Webster, D., & Nopp, P. (2005). Investigations into electrically evoked stapedius reflex measures and subjective loudness percepts in the MED-EL COMBI 40+ cochlear implant. *Cochlear Implants International, 6*(1), 31–42.

Brown, C. J., Abbas, P. J., Fryauf-Bertschy, H., Kelsay, D., & Gantz, B. J. (1994). Intraoperative and postoperative electrically evoked auditory brain stem responses in nucleus cochlear implant users: Implications for the fitting process. *Ear and Hearing, 15*(2), 168–176.

Buchman, C. A., Copeland, B. J., Yu, K. K., Brown, C. J., Carrasco, V. N., & Pillsbury III, H. C. (2004). Cochlear implantation in children with congenital inner ear malformations. *Laryngoscope, 114*(2), 309–316.

Buchman, C. A., Roush, P. A., Teagle, H. F., Brown, C. J., Zdanski, C. J., & Grose, J. H. (2006). Auditory neuropathy characteristics in children with cochlear nerve deficiency. *Ear and Hearing, 27*(40), 399–408.

Buchner A., Frohne-Buchner, C., Battmer, R., & Lenarz, T. (2004) Two years of experience using stimulation rates between 800 and 5000 pps with the Clarion CI implant. *International Congress Series, 1273*, 48–51.

Buchner, A., Nogueira, W., Edler, B., Battmer, R., & Lenarz, T. (2008). Results from a psychoacoustic model-based strategy for the Nucleus-24 and Freedom cochlear implants. *Otology and Neurotology, 29*, 189–192.

Buckler, L., & Overstreet, E. (2003). *Relationship between electrical stapedial reflex thresholds and Hi-Res program settings: Potential tool for pediatric cochlear-implant fitting.* Valencia, CA: Advanced Bionics.

Carhart, R., & Jerger, J. F. (1959). Preferred method for clinical determination of pure-tone thresholds. *Journal of Speech and Hearing Disorders, 24*, 330–345.

Ching, T. Y., Psarros, C., Hill, M., Dillon, H., & Incerti, P. (2001). Should children who use cochlear implants wear hearing aids in the opposite ear? *Ear and Hearing, 22*(5), 365–380.

Ching, T. Y., Incerti, P., & Hill, M. (2004). Binaural benefits for adults who use hearing aids and cochlear implants in opposite ears. *Ear and Hearing, 25*(1), 9–21.

Cochlear Corporation (2008, June). *Nucleus Reliability Report, 5*, 1–8. Retrieved October 8, 2009, from http://professionals.cochlearamericas.com/sites/default/files/resources/N33357F_ISS1_JUNE08_Reliablility_Report_AQM.pdf

Dawson, P., Skok, M., & Clark, G. (1997). The effect of loudness imbalance between electrodes in cochlear implant users. *Ear and Hearing, 18*, 156–165.

Dawson, P. W., Decker, J. A., & Psarros, C. E. (2004). Optimizing dynamic range in children using the Nucleus cochlear implant. *Ear and Hearing, 25*(3), 230–241.

Dorman, M., Loizou, P., Spahr, A., & Maloff, E. (2002). A comparison of the speech understanding provided by acoustic models of fixed-channel and channel-picking signal processors for cochlear implants. *Journal of Speech, Language, and Hearing Research, 45*(4), 783–788.

Dorman, M., & Dahlstrom, L., (2004). Speech understanding by cochlear-implant patients with different left- and right-ear electrode arrays. *Ear and Hearing, 25*(2), 191–194.

Dunn, C., Tyler, R., Witt, S., & Gantz, B. (2006). Effects of converting bilateral cochlear implant subjects to a strategy with increased rate and number of channels. *Annals of Otology, Rhinology, and Laryngology, 115*(6), 425—432.

Durisin, M., Arnoldner, C., Stover, T., Lenarz, T., & Lesinski-Schiedat, A. (2008). Audiological performance in cochlear implanted patients deafened by meningitis depending on duration of deafness. *European Archives of Otorhinolaryngology, 265*(4), 381–388.

Fetterman, B. L., & Domico, E. H. (2002). Speech recognition in background noise of cochlear implant patients. *Otolaryngology–Head & Neck Surgery, 126*(3), 257–263.

Finley, C. C., Holden, T. A., Holden, L. K., Whiting, B. R., Chole, R. A., Neely, G. J., . . . Skinner, M. W. (2008). Role of electrode placement as a contributor to variability in cochlear implant outcomes. *Otology and Neurotology, 29*(7), 920–928.

Firszt, J. B., Holden, L. K., Skinner, M. W., Tobey, E. A., Peterson, A., Gaggl, W., Samuelson, C. L., & Wackym, P. A. (2004). Recognition of speech presented at soft to loud levels by adult cochlear implant recipients of three cochlear implant systems. *Ear and Hearing, 25*(4), 375–387.

Franck, K. (2002) A model of a Nucleus 24 cochlear implant fitting protocol based on the electrically evoked whole nerve potential. *Ear and Hearing, 23*(1), 67S–71S.

Geers, A., Brenner, C., & Davidson, L. (2004). Factors associated with development of speech perception skills in children implanted by age five. *Ear and Hearing, 24*(Suppl. 1), 24S–35S.

Geers, A. E. (2004). Speech, language, and reading skills after early cochlear implantation. *Archives of Otolaryngology–Head & Neck Surgery, 130*(5), 634–638.

Geers, A. E., Moog, J. S., Biedenstein, J., Brenner, C., & Hayes, H. (2009). Spoken language scores of children using cochlear implants compared to hearing age-mates at school entry. *Journal of Deaf Studies and Deaf Education, 14*(3), 371–385.

Gibson, W. P., Sanli, H., & Psarros, C. (2009). The use of intra-operative electrical auditory brainstem responses to predict the speech perception outcome after cochlear implantation *Cochlear Implants International, 10*(Suppl. 1), 52–57.

Gifford, R. H., Shallop, J. K., & Peterson, A. M. (2008). Speech recognition materials and ceiling effects: Considerations for cochlear implant programs. *Audiology and Neurotology, 13*(3), 193–205.

Gifford, R. G., & Revit, U. (2010). *Speech perception for cochlear implant recipients in a realistic background noise: Effectiveness of preprocessing strategies and external options for improving sentence recognition in noise.* Manuscript submitted for publication.

Gordon, K. A., Papsin, B. C., & Harrison, R. V. (2004). Toward a battery of behavioral and objective measures to achieve optimal cochlear implant stimulation levels in children. *Ear and Hearing, 25*(5), 447–463.

Green, K. M., Bhatt, Y. M., Mawman, D. J., O'Driscoll, M. P., Saeed, S. R., Ramsden, R. T., & Green, M. W. (2007). Predictors of audiological outcome following cochlear implantation in adults. *Cochlear Implants International, 8*(1), 1–11.

Hamzavi, J., Baumgartner, W. D., Pok, S. M., Franz, P., & Gstoettner, W. (2003). Variables affecting speech perception in postlingually deaf adults following cochlear implantation. *Acta Otolaryngologica, 123*(4), 493–498.

Helms, J., Weichbold, V., Baumann, U., von Specht, H., Schon, F., Muller, J., . . . D'Haese, P. (2004). Analysis of ceiling effects occurring with speech recognition tests in adult cochlear-implanted patients. *Journal for Oto-Rhino-Laryngology and Its Related Specialties, 66*(3), 130–135.

Henkin, Y., Kaplan-Neeman, R., Muchnik, C., Kronenberg, J., & Hildesheimer, M. (2003). Changes over time in electrical stimulation levels and electrode impedance values in children using the Nucleus 24M cochlear implant. *International Journal of Pediatric Otorhinolaryngology, 67*(8), 873–880.

Henkin, Y., Kaplan-Neeman, R., Kronenberg, J., Migirov, L., Hildesheimer, M., & Muchnik, C. (2006). A longitudinal study of electrical stimulation levels and electrode impedance in children using the Clarion cochlear implant. *Acta Otolaryngologica, 126*(6), 581–586.

Hodges, A. V., Balkany, T. J., Ruth, R. A., Lambert, P. R., Dolan-Ash, S., & Schloffman, J. J. (1997). Electrical middle ear muscle reflex: use in cochlear implant programming. *Otolaryngology–Head & Neck Surgery, 117*(3 Pt 1), 255–261.

Hughes, M., Brown, C., Abbas, P., Wolaver A., & Gervais, J. (2000). Comparison of EAP thresholds with MAP levels in the Nucleus 24 cochlear implant: Data from children. *Ear and Hearing, 21*(2), 164–174.

Hughes, M. L., Vander Werff, K. R., Brown, C. J., Abbas, P. J., Kelsay, D. M., Teagle, H. F., & Lowder, M. W. (2001). A longitudinal study of electrode impedance, the electrically evoked compound action potential, and behavioral measures in Nucleus 24 cochlear implant users. *Ear and Hearing, 22*(6), 471–486.

James, C. J., Blamey, P. J., Martin, L., Swanson, B., Just, Y., & Macfarlane, D. (2002). Adaptive dynamic range optimization for cochlear implants: A preliminary study. *Ear and Hearing, 23*(Suppl. 1), 49S–58S.

Jeong, S. W., Kim, L. S., Kim, B. Y., Bae, W. Y., & Kim, J. R. (2007). Cochlear implantation in children with auditory neuropathy: outcomes and rationale. *Acta Otolaryngologica Supplementum, 558*, 36–43.

Jerger, J., Oliver, T. A., & Chmiel, R. A. (1988). Prediction of dynamic range from stapedius reflex in cochlear implant patients. *Ear and Hearing. 9*(1), 4–8.

Kaplan, D. M., Shipp, D. B., Chen, J. M., Ng, A. H., & Nedzelski, J. M. (2003). Early-deafened adult cochlear implant users: assessment of outcomes. *Journal of Otolaryngology, 32*(4), 245–249.

Kiefer, J., Hohl, S., Sturzebecher, E., Pfennigdorff, T., & Gstöettner, W. (2001). Comparison of speech recognition with different speech coding strategies (SPEAK, CIS, and ACE) and their relationship to telemetric measures of compound action potentials in the nucleus CI 24M cochlear implant system. *Audiology, 40*(1), 32–42.

Kileny, P. R., & Zwolan, T.A. (2004). Pre-perioperative, transtympanic electrically evoked auditory brainstem response in children. *International Journal of Audiology,* (Suppl. 1), S16–21.

Kileny, P. R. (2007). Evoked potentials in the management of patients with cochlear implants: Research and clinical applications. *Ear and Hearing,* (Suppl. 2), 124S–127S.

Koch, D. B., Osberger, M. J., Segel, P., & Kessler, D. K. (2004). HiResolution and conventional sound processing in the HiResolution Bionic Ear: using appropriate outcome measures to assess speech-recognition ability. *Audiology and Neurotology, 9*, 214–223.

Lane, J. I., Driscoll, C. L., Witte, R. J., Primak, A., & Lindell, E. P. (2007). Scalar localization of the electrode array after cochlear implantation: A cadaveric validation study comparing 64 slice multidetector computed tomography with microcomputed tomography. *Otology and Neurotology, 28*(2), 191–194.

Ling, D. (1976). *Speech and the hearing-impaired child: Theory and Practice.* Washington, DC: Alexander Graham Bell Association for the Deaf.

Ling, D. (1989). *Foundations of spoken language for the hearing-impaired child.* Washington, DC: Alexander Graham Bell Association for the Deaf.

Lorens, A., Walkowiak, A., Piotrowska, A., Skarzynski, H., & Anderson, I. (2004). ESRT and MCL correlations in experienced paediatric cochlear implant users. *Cochlear Implants International, 5*(1), 28–37.

Loundon, N., Rouillon, I., Munier, N., Marlin, S., Roger, G., & Garabedian, E. N. (2005). Cochlear implantation in children with internal ear malformations. *Otology and Neurotology, 26*(4), 668–673.

Madell, J. R. (2008). Using behavioral observation audiometry to evaluate hearing in infants from birth to six months. In J. R. Madell & C. Flexer (Eds.), *Pediatric audiology: Diagnosis, technology, and management* (pp. 54–63). New York, NY: Thieme Medical.

Manrique, M., Huarte, A., Morera, C., Caballe, L., Ramos, A., Castillo, C., . . . Juan, E. (2005). Speech perception with the ACE and the SPEAK speech coding strategies for children implanted with the Nucleus cochlear implant. *International Journal of Pediatric Otorhinolaryngology, 69*(12), 1667–1674.

MED-EL Corporation. (2009, July). Retrieved October 8, 2009, from http://www.medel.com/english/img/animations/SONATA_CSR.swf

Migirov, L., Taitelbaum-Swead, R., Drendel, M., Hildesheimer, M., & Kronenberg, J. (2009). Cochlear implantation in elderly patients: Surgical and audiological outcome. *Gerontology*. Retrieved October 1, 2009, from http://content.karger.com/ProdukteDB/produkte.asp?typ=pdf&doi=235864

Mitchell, T. E., Psarros, C., Pegg, P., Rennie, M., & Gibson, W. P. (2000). Performance after cochlear implantation: A comparison of children deafened by meningitis and congenitally deaf children. *Journal of Laryngology and Otology, 114*(1), 33–37.

Moller, A. (2001). Neurophysiologic basis for cochlear and auditory brainstem implants. *American Journal of Audiology, 10*(2), 68–77.

Moller, A. (2006). Physiological basis for cochlear and auditory brainstem implants. *Advances in Otorhinolaryngology, 64*, 206–223.

Moore, B. C. (2003). Coding of sounds in the auditory system and its relevance in signal processing and coding in cochlear implants. *Otology and Neurotology, 24*(2), 243–254.

Müller-Deile, J., Kiefer, J., Wyss, J., Nicolai, J., & Battmer, R. (2008). Performance benefits for adults using a cochlear implant with adaptive dynamic range optimization (ADRO): A comparative study. *Cochlear Implants International, 9*(1), 8–26.

Mylanus, E. A., Rotteveel, L. J., & Leeuw, R. L. (2004). Congenital malformation of the inner ear and pediatric cochlear implantation. *Otology and Neurotology, 25*(3), 308–317.

Nelson, D., Schmitz, J., Donaldson, G., Viemeister, N., & Javel, E. (1996). Intensity discrimination as a function of stimulus level with electric stimulation. *Journal of the Acoustical Society of America, 100*(4 Pt. 1), 2393–2414.

Nicholas, J. G., & Geers, A. E. (2007). Will they catch up? The role of age at cochlear implantation in the spoken language development of children with severe to profound hearing loss. *Journal of Speech, Language, and Hearing Research, 50*(4), 1048–1062.

Nilsson, M., Soli, S. D., & Sullivan, J. A. (1994). Development of the Hearing in Noise Test for the measurement of speech reception thresholds in quiet and in noise. *Journal of the Acoustical Society of America, 95*(2), 1085–1099.

Noble, W., Tyler R. S., Dunn, C. C., & Bhullar, N. (2009). Younger- and older-age adults with unilateral and bilateral cochlear implants: Speech and spatial hearing self-ratings and performance. *Otology & Neurotology, 30*(7), 921–929.

Oh, S. H., Kim, C. S., Kang, E. J., Lee, D. S., Lee, H. J., Chang, S. O., . . . Koo, J. W. (2003). Speech perception after cochlear implantation over a 4-year time period. *Acta Otolaryngologica, 23*(2), 148–153.

Pasanisi, E., Bacciu, A., Vincenti, V., Guida, M., Berghenti, M. T., Barbot, A., . . . Bacciu, S. (2002). Comparison of speech perception benefits with SPEAK and ACE coding strategies in pediatric Nucleus CI24M cochlear implant recipients. *International Journal of Pediatric Otorhinolaryngology, 64*(2), 159–163.

Peterson, A., Shallop, J., Driscoll, C., Breneman, A., Babb, J., Stoeckel, R., & Fabry, L. (2003). Outcomes of cochlear implantation in children with auditory neuropathy. *Journal of the American Academy of Audiology, 14*(4), 188–201.

Plant, K., Law, M. A., Whitford, L., Knight, M., Tari, S., Leigh, J., . . . Nel, E. (2005). Evaluation of streamlined programming procedures for the Nucleus cochlear implant with the Contour electrode array. *Ear and Hearing, 26*(6), 651–668.

Postnov, A., Zarowski, A., De Clerck, N., Vanpoucke, F., Offeciers, F. E., Van Dyck, D., & Peeters, S. (2006). High resolution micro-CT scanning as an innovative tool for evaluation of the surgical positioning of cochlear implant electrodes. *Acta Otolaryngologica, 126*(5), 467–474.

Rance, G. (2005). Auditory neuropathy/dys-synchrony and its perceptual consequences. *Trends in Amplification, 9*(1), 1–43.

Rance, G., & Barker, E. J. (2008). Speech perception in children with auditory neuropathy/dyssynchrony managed with either hearing aids or cochlear implants. *Otology and Neurotology, 29*(2), 179–182.

Robbins, A. M. (2005). Clinical Red Flags for slow progress in children with cochlear implants. In *Loud and Clear 1*. Valencia, CA: Advanced Bionics.

Sainz, M., de la Torre, A., Roldan, C., Ruiz, J., & Vargas, J. (2003). Analysis of programming maps and its application for balancing multichannel cochlear implants. *International Journal of Audiology, 42*(1), 43–51.

Santarelli, R., De Filippi, R., Genovese, E., & Arslan, E. (2008). Cochlear implantation outcome in prelingually deafened young adults. A speech perception study. *Audiology and Neuro-otology, 13*(4), 257–265.

Schafer, E. C., & Thibodeau, L. M. (2004). Speech recognition abilities of adults using cochlear implants interfaced with FM systems. *Journal of the American Academy of Audiology, 15*(10), 678–691.

Schafer, E. C., Amlani, A. M., Seibold, A., & Shattuck, P. L. (2007). A meta-analytic comparison of binaural benefits between bilateral cochlear implants and bimodal stimulation. *Journal of the American Academy of Audiology, 18*(9), 760–776.

Schafer, E. C., Wolfe, J., Lawless, T., & Stout, B. (2009). Effects of FM-receiver gain on speech-recognition performance of adults with cochlear implants. *International Journal of Audiology, 48*(4), 196–203.

Schafer, E. C. & Kleineck, M. P. (in press). Improvements in speech-recognition performance using cochlear implants and three types of FM systems: A meta-analytic approach. *Journal of Educational Audiology, 15.*

Serpanos, Y. & Gravel, J. (2002). Growth of loudness assessment in children using cross-modality matching (CMM). In R. Seewald & J. Gravel (Eds.), *A Sound Foundation Through Early Amplification, Proceedings of the Second International Conference* (pp. 75–84). Switzerland: Phonak AG.

Sharma, A., & Dorman, M.F. (2006). Central auditory development in children with cochlear implants: Clinical implications. *Advances in Otorhinolaryngology, 64*, 66–88.

Skinner, M., Holden, L., Holden, T. (1994). Effect of frequency boundary assignment on speech recognition with the Speak speech-coding strategy. *Annals of Otology, Rhinology, and Laryngology, 104*(Suppl. 166), 307–311.

Skinner, M. W., Holden, L. K., Holden, T. A. (1995). Effect of frequency boundary assignment on speech recognition with the SPEAK speech-coding strategy. *Annals of Otology, Rhinology, and Laryngology, 104*(Suppl. 166), 307–311.

Skinner, M. W., Holden, L. K., Holden, T. A., Demorest, M.E. (1995). Comparison of procedures for obtaining thresholds and maximum acceptable loudness levels with the Nucleus Cochlear Implant System. *Journal of Speech and Hearing Research, 38*, 677–689.

Skinner, M. W., Holden, L. K., Holden, T. A. (1997). Parameter selection to optimize speech recognition with the Nucleus implant. *Otolaryngology-Head and Neck Surgery, 117*(3 Pt 1), 188–195.

Skinner, M. W., Holden, L. K., Holden, T. A., & Demorest, M. E. (1999). Comparison of two methods for selecting minimum stimulation levels used in programming the Nucleus 22 cochlear implant. *Journal of Speech, Language, and Hearing Research, 42*(4), 814–828.

Skinner, M. W., Holden, L. K., Whitford, L. A., Plant, K. L., Psarros, C., & Holden, T. A. (2002). Speech recognition with the nucleus 24 SPEAK, ACE, and CIS speech coding strategies in newly implanted adults. *Ear and Hearing, 23*(3), 207–223.

Spahr, A. J., & Dorman, M. F. (2005). Effects of minimum stimulation settings for the Med El Tempo+ speech processor on speech understanding. *Ear and Hearing, 26*(Suppl. 4), 2S–6S.

Spahr, A. J., Dorman, M. F., & Loiselle, L. H. (2007). Performance of patients using different cochlear implant systems: Effect of input dynamic range. *Ear and Hearing, 28*(2), 260–275.

Spivak, L. G., & Chute, P. M. (1994). The relationship between electrical acoustic reflex thresholds and behavioral comfort levels in children and adult cochlear implant patients. *Ear and Hearing, 15*(2), 184–192.

Spivak, L. G., Chute, P. M., Popp, A. L., & Parisier, S. C. (1994). Programming the cochlear implant based on electrical acoustic reflex thresholds: patient performance. *Laryngoscope, 104*(10), 1225–1230.

Spriet, A., Van Deun, L., Eftaxiadis, K., Laneau, J., Moonen, M., van Dijk, B., . . . Wouters, J. (2007). Speech understanding in background noise with the two-microphone adaptive beamformer BEAM in the Nucleus Freedom Cochlear Implant System. *Ear and Hearing, 28*(1), 62–72.

Stelmachowicz, P. G., Pittman, A. L., Hoover, B. M., & Lewis, D. E. (2001). Effect of stimulus bandwidth on the perception of /s/ in normal- and hearing-impaired children and adults. *Journal of the Acoustical Society of America, 110*(4), 2183–2190.

Teoh, S. W., Pisoni, D. B., & Miyamoto, R. T. (2004). Cochlear implantation in adults with prelingual deafness. Part I. Clinical results. *Laryngoscope, 114*(9), 1536–1540.

Tyler, R., Dunn, C., Witt, S., Noble, W., Gantz, B., Rubinstein, J., . . . Litovsky, R. (2006). Soundfield hearing for patients with cochlear implants and hearing aids. In H. Cooper & L. Craddock (Eds.), *Cochlear implants: A practical guide.* West Sussex, UK: Whurr.

Vandali, A., Whitford, L., Plant, K., & Clark, G. (2000). Speech perception as a function of electrical stimulation rate: using the Nucleus 24 cochlear implant system. *Ear and Hearing, 21*, 608–624.

Walton, J., Gibson, W.P., Sanli, H., & Prelog, K. (2008). Predicting cochlear implant outcomes in children with auditory neuropathy. *Otology and Neurotology, 29*(3), 302–309.

Wier, C., Jesteadt, W., & Green, D. M. (1977). Frequency discrimination as a function of frequency and sensation level. *Journal of the Acoustical Society of America, 61,* 178–184.

Wolfe, J., Baker, S., Caraway, T., Kasulis, H., Mears, A., Smith, J., . . . Wood, M. (2007). One-year post activation results for sequentially implanted bilateral cochlear implant users. *Otology and Neurotology, 28*(5), 589–596.

Wolfe, J., & Kasulis, H. (2008). Relationships among objective measures and speech perception in adult users of the HiResolution Bionic Ear. *Cochlear Implants International, 9*(2), 70–81.

Wolfe, J. & Schafer, E. C. (2008). Evaluation of the iConnect FM adapter in children. In *Auditory research bulletin: 2007 biennial edition* (pp. 120–121). Valencia, CA: Advanced Bionics.

Wolfe, J., & Schafer, E. C. (2008). Optimizing the benefits of Auria sound processors coupled to personal FM systems with iConnect adaptors. *Journal of the American Academy of Audiology, 19*(8), 585–594.

Wolfe, J., Schafer, E. C., Heldner, B., Mulder, H., Ward, E., & Vincent, B. (2009). Evaluation of speech recognition in noise with cochlear implants and Dynamic FM. *Journal of the American Academy of Audiology, 20*(7), 409–421.

Zeitler, D. M., Budenz, C. L. & Roland Jr., J. T. (2009). Revision cochlear implantation. *CurrentOpinion in Otolaryngology & Head and Neck Surgery, 17*(5), 334–338.

Zeng, F., & Galvin, J. (1999). Amplitude mapping and phoneme recognition in cochlear implant listeners. *Ear and Hearing, 20*(1), 60–74.

Zwolan, T., Kileny, P., Smith, S., Mills, D., Koch, D, & Osberger, M. (2001). Adult cochlear implant performance with evolving electrode technology. *Otology and Neurotology, 22*(6), 844–849.

Zwolan T. & Overstreet, E. (2005). Setting upper program levels in children. In *Auditory research bulletin: Biennial edition 2005* (pp. 54–56). Valencia, CA: Advanced Bionics.

Zwolan, T. A., O'Sullivan, M. B., Fink, N. E., Niparko, J. K., & The CDACI Investigative Team. (2008). Electric charge requirements of pediatric cochlear implant recipients enrolled in the childhood development after cochlear implantation study. *Otology and Neurotology, 29,* 143–148.

Index

Note: Numbers in **bold** reference non-text material.